HOMEMADE KETO SOUP COOKBOOK

Fat Burning & Delicious Soups, Stews, Broths & Bread.

Low-carb comfort food for the soul.

Elizabeth Jane

INTRODUCTION

I have created this book in hopes of inspiring you to make soup a staple in your ketogenic diet and to enjoy the simplicity of making them. Since starting my keto journey, I have learned to love soups as they are something I can throw together in my Instant Pot or slow cooker quickly and add a ton of nourishing ingredients into one recipe. I also love the versatility of making soup, which is what I have tried to offer in this book. I wanted to cater to as many different dietary needs as I could by providing 100% gluten-free recipes with some vegetarian and meat-based options as well.

You will also find homemade broths and a large variety of different soup options to fit everyone's flavor preferences. Here, you'll find from creamy soups to bisques, chowders, chilis, homemade broths and even some cleansing cold soup options for those who are looking for lighter and more refreshing soup options.

I hope you find some inspiration in this book and take advantage of just how easy and delicious making homemade soup can be. I also hope you find a recipe for every season of the year as soup doesn't only have to be for the colder months! Making soup a regular part of your ketogenic diet all year long is an excellent way to support overall health and makes meal prep that much easier.

TABLE OF CONTENTS

L = <30% calories from fat,
M = 30%-59% calories from fat,
H = >60% calories from fat

Vegetarian Soups

Creamy Soups

**L = <30% calories from fat,
M = 30%-59% calories from fat,
H = >60% calories from fat**

Spicy Soups

Cold Soups

Quick & Easy Soups-5 Ingredients or Less

L = **<30% calories from fat,**
M = **30%-59% calories from fat,**
H = **>60% calories from fat**

Vegetarian Comfort Stews

Meat-Based Comfort Stews

Side Dishes

**L = <30% calories from fat,
M = 30%-59% calories from fat,
H = >60% calories from fat**

Bisques, Chowders and Broths

Soup Bread

Soup Seasonings & Toppings

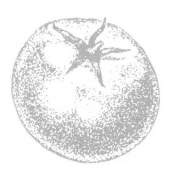

L = <30% calories from fat,
M = 30%-59% calories from fat,
H = >60% calories from fat

MAKING THE PERFECT SOUP

I want to kick things off by talking about how to make perfect soups and broths. This is a general guide of mixing ingredients for the perfect flavor, simmer and cook times and some general tips that I have found helpful along the way.

Best Flavor Combinations for Soup

Depending on what type of soup you are going for, I have come up with a guide with some of my personal favorite flavor combinations. These spices tend to pair well together and make for a very flavorful soup.

Carrots + Ginger + Turmeric

Avocado + Cilantro + Lime + Sea Salt

Walnuts + Cheese + Nutmeg

Garlic + Tomato+ Onion

Cucumbers + Fresh Herbs

Cayenne Pepper + Cinnamon

Mozzarella Cheese + Tomato + Basil

Pumpkin + Butter + Bone Broth + Sage

Lemon + Chicken + Fennel

Pine Nuts + Basil + Feta Cheese

Fish + Lemon + Fennel

Do you have to brown ground beef before adding it to your slow cooker?

To save yourself some time and added cleanup, try using lean ground beef in your recipe to prevent having to brown the beef before adding it to your slow cooker. If you are unable to find lean ground beef, brown the beef and then drain the grease before adding it to the slow cooker.

How to Make a Creamy Soup

Many of the soups in this book contain heavy cream or coconut milk for a vegetarian version. To make a delicious creamy soup, you will want to add the cream after the soup has finished cooking, and be sure to warm the cream first. Adding cold cream will curdle if added to a hot soup.

Simmering the Perfect Soup & Broth

Once you bring your soup to a boil, you will want to reduce it to a simmer. Boiling the soup for the entire cooking time can make for mushy veggies!

General Tricks of the Soup & Broth Cooking Trade

- Double or triple your recipes to freeze for later use.
- Divide the soup into single servings before freezing to take out and enjoy as a quick meal when you don't have time to meal prep.
- Chop up your veggies into bite-sized pieces. You don't want large chunks in each spoonful,
- Season your soup or broth after you cook it so you can adjust the taste accordingly.
- Use an immersion blender when needed if you are looking for a smooth soup. You can cook all of the ingredients together, and then blend once cooked.

Tips for substituting greens

Greens can be a personal choice but can be easily swapped for another variety.

Do not like kale? Try substituting it for spinach (better to be regular spinach than baby spinach) or Swiss/rainbow chard can work as well, too.

Greens can handle long cooking times like kale; spinach and chard should be added right before serving on the last few minutes of cooking.

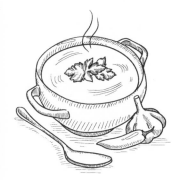

HOW TO MAKE SOUP IN AN INSTANT POT OR SLOW COOKER

I wanted to briefly touch upon making soup in an Instant Pot or a slow cooker to give you that option. Each of the recipes can be made in either one depending on your preference. You can also simmer your soups or stews. On days where I have a little extra time, I choose to simmer my soups on the stove. However, on days where my time is limited, I will choose to use my Instant Pot or slow cooker. It all comes down to preference, and I always find it's better to have options.

A General Guide to Using an Instant Pot to Make Soup

The Instant Pot has an actual soup setting, which makes things easy. You can cook your soup anywhere from 20 minutes to 50 minutes. There is also a meat or stew setting, which will make your meat fall right off the bone. It is so easy to use!

I like to use the Instant Pot when I am cooking heavily meat-based soups and stews as it makes the meat extremely tender and brings the flavors together nicely.

A General Guide to Using a Slow Cooker to Make Soup

You can also use a slow cooker to cook your soups or stews. In fact, many of the recipes in this book recommend that you cook your soup in a slow cooker. If you have an Instant Pot, you can also use the slow cooker setting.

As a general rule, you can toss all of the ingredients into the base of a slow cooker (except cream or other dairy products) and cook on high for 3 to 4 hours or low for 6 to 8 hours. If you are adding heavy cream, cream cheese, sour cream or any other dairy product, you can do so at the end. However, always warm milk and heavy cream before adding it to a hot soup.

Weights:

Throughout the book we have consistent weights for ingredients, however you may struggle to find the exact same weight, e.g. it might be hard for you to find a chicken breast exactly 4 oz.

I would encourage you to not over-complicate recipes and purchase 'average pieces' of such ingredients, rather than specific pieces. For reference below are the weights we constantly use throughout the book:

Chicken breast (boneless): 4 ounces

Carrot: 2.2 ounces

Yellow onion: 8 ounces

Avocado: 6 ounces

Cucumber: 11 ounces

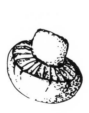

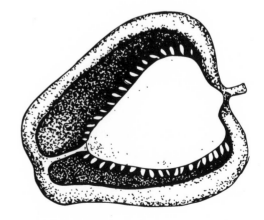

HOW TO STORE YOUR SOUP

Batch cooking soups and stews is an excellent way to save you time and energy during the busy work week. You can double or triple your recipes easily and freeze individual portions for later use.

I love to freeze individual soup portions in silicone freezer trays, and then label them in the freezer. This makes it super easy to pop out single servings and reheat for a quick and nourishing meal.

It's best to freeze any soup you won't be enjoying within a couple of days. When it comes time to reheat, you can add the soup to a stockpot over low to medium heat until defrosted and warmed through.

You can also make a big batch of homemade broth and freeze it the same way. When you are ready to make your homemade soup, you can pop the broth out of the silicone trays and defrost it on the stove.

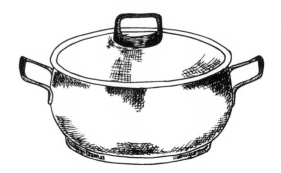

MUST-HAVE COOKING UTENSILS FOR THE PERFECT SOUP

Over the years, I have found a handful of kitchen tools that make cooking so much easier! I wanted to put together a list of my favorite cooking utensils to help you make the perfect soup. These are staples in my kitchen and some of my best investments because they can be used for dozens of different recipes.

Instant Pot: In this next section of this book, I talk about how much I love my Instant Pot! I love to make soups and stews in it, and it makes cleanup so much easier.

http://ketojane.com/instantpot

Immersion Blender: An immersion blender is a must in my kitchen! It makes blending soup so much easier and prevents me from having to pour the entire soup recipe into my blender. I personally like this Cuisinart model.

http://ketojane.com/blender

Silicone Freezer Cubes: I love these for soup! I try to avoid plastic as much as possible, and these make freezing smaller individual portions of soup so much easier. I can pop out a single serving and defrost as needed.

http://ketojane.com/cubes

Silicone Soup Ladle: This is my favorite soup ladle. It makes portioning out homemade soup easy, and it scoops out a decent amount of soup, so you don't have to worry about soup spilling everywhere.

http://ketojane.com/ladle

Spice Containers: These spice containers are perfect for making your own spice mixes. You can place them in these glass jars and label them so you can see what spices you have to add to your soups and stews. They are also cute, so they will blend in with most kitchen décor.

http://ketojane.com/spice

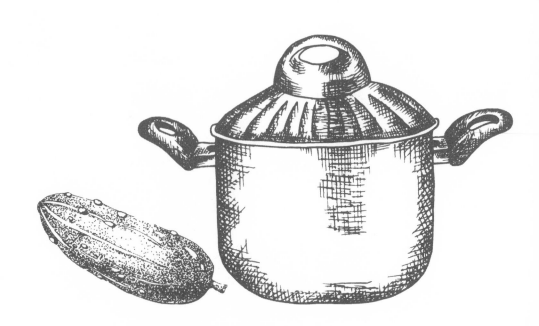

BONUS KETO SWEET EATS

I am delighted you have chosen my book to help you start or continue on your keto journey. Temptation by sweet treats can knock you off course so, to help you stay on the keto track, I am pleased to offer you three mini ebooks from my 'Keto Sweet Eats Series', completely free of charge! These three mini ebooks cover how to make everything from keto chocolate cake to keto ice cream to keto fat bombs so you don't have to feel like you are missing out, whatever the occasion.

Simply visit the link below to get your free copy of all three mini ebooks:

http://ketojane.com/saucebonus

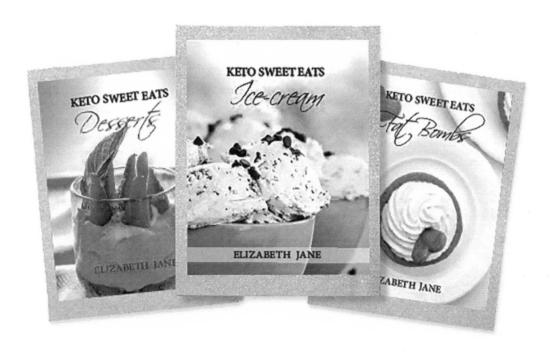

HOW THIS BOOK WORKS

This cookbook contains helpful cooking tips to help you get the best results possible. There are also serving suggestions included to give you an idea about what each of these recipes pairs well with.

You will also notice there are five symbols on the top right-hand side of each recipe. A key to these symbols is set out below:

Preparation Time:

The time required to prepare the recipe. This does not include the cooking time.

Cooking Time:

The time required to cook the recipe. This does not include the preparation time.

Servings:

The number of servings each recipe provides. This can be adjusted. For example, by doubling the quantity of all of the ingredients, you can make twice as many servings.

Difficulty Level:

1: An easy-to-make recipe that can be put together with just a handful of ingredients and in a short amount of time.

2: These recipes are a little more difficult and time-consuming but are still easy enough — even for beginners!

3: A more advanced recipe for the adventurous cook! You will not see too many Level 3 recipes in this book. These recipes are ideal for when you have a bit more time to spend in the kitchen and when you want to make something out of the ordinary.

Cost:

$: A low-budget, everyday recipe.

$$: A moderately priced, middle-of-the-road recipe.

$$$: A more expensive recipe that is great for serving at a family gathering or party. These recipes tend to contain pricey ingredients.

Keto-Meter

This is something new that I have decided to include as I think it will be a great way to help you determine where each recipe stands on my custom made keto-meter. This will give you a better idea as far as how keto the recipe is vs. how low carb the recipe is. I use calories from fat (%) to determine how keto each recipe is. You will see a label on each recipe indicating if a recipe falls within the low, medium, or high category.

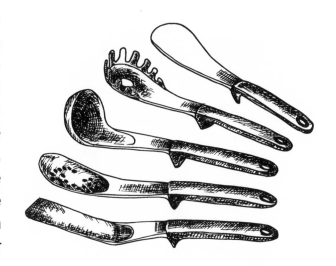

Keto-meter key:

 <30% calories from fats

 31-60% calories from fats

 >61% calories from fats

In the index contents page these are

L = <30% calories from fat,

M = 30%-59% calories from fat,

H = >60% calories from fat

Dietary Labels

V: Vegetarian : Vegetarian recipes are meat-free, but may still contain some dairy products like heavy cream or cheese. If you need to avoid dairy, you can eliminate the cheese or choose a low-calorie, nut-based cheese, and you can swap out the heavy cream for full-fat coconut milk.

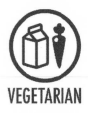

VEGETARIAN

YOU MAY ALSO LIKE

Please visit the below link, for another books by the author

http://ketojane.com/books

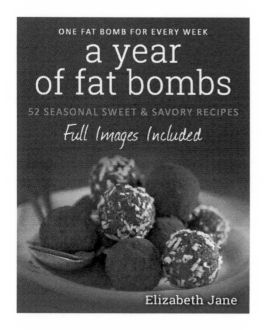

The seasons change, and so do your fat-burning keto treats. Energize yourself all year round with sweet and savory goodness.

52 delicious seasonal recipes keep you in ketosis when you feel the need to snack.

⭐⭐⭐⭐½ ▾   70 customer reviews

A Year of Fat Bombs: 52 Seasonal Sweet & Savory Recipes

Perfect to make ahead and snack on to the go.

Visit the link below to get your copy.

http://ketojane.com/bombs

On a keto or low-carb diet and miss bread? Then this book is for you.

Do you want to use fat to fuel your body? Do you want to stop counting calories forever?

The **"Ultimate Keto Diet Guide"** shows you how to tailor the keto diet to your lifestyle along with 100 delicious fat burning recipes.

Visit the link below to get your copy

http://ketojane.com/burn

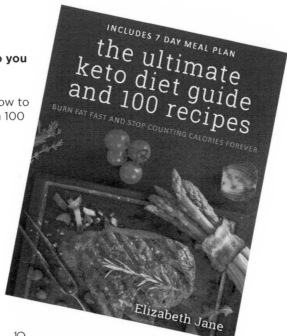

FINAL WORDS

Finally, I want to thank you for purchasing this book, and I hope it helps you keep to your health goals.

If you enjoyed this book or have any suggestions, then I would love it if you would be kind enough to leave a review (on the link below) or simply email me (I personally answer all emails).

elizabeth@ketojane.com

To leave a review on Amazon, please visit:
http://ketojane.com/reviewmysoup

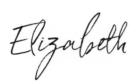

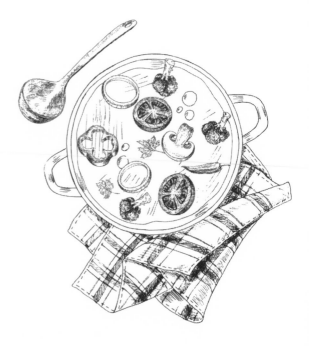

Meat-Based Soups

THYME & BASIL BEEF SOUP (M)

MEDIUM

Serves: 6

Prep Time: 15 minutes

Cook Time: 40 minutes

Difficulty Level: 1

Cost: $$

Calories: 219
Carbs: 6g
Fiber: 1g
Net Carbs: 5g
Fat: 9g
Protein: 29g

Calories from:
Carbs: 9%
Fats: 37%
Protein: 53%

Ingredients:

- 1 pound beef chuck roast, cubed
- 6 cups beef bone broth (you can also use regular beef broth)
- 1 yellow onion, chopped
- 2 cloves garlic, chopped
- 2 carrots, chopped
- 2 stalks celery, sliced
- 1 teaspoon fresh thyme, chopped
- ½ teaspoon dried oregano
- 1 handful fresh basil, chopped
- Salt & pepper, to taste
- 1 tablespoon coconut oil, for cooking

Directions:

1. Add the coconut oil to a skillet and brown the beef over medium heat.

2. Add the beef and the remaining ingredients minus the basil to a stockpot and bring to a boil.

3. Reduce to a simmer and cook for about 30 minutes or until the vegetables are tender.

4. Serve with freshly chopped basil.

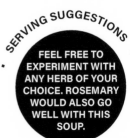

SERVING SUGGESTIONS

FEEL FREE TO EXPERIMENT WITH ANY HERB OF YOUR CHOICE. ROSEMARY WOULD ALSO GO WELL WITH THIS SOUP.

GARLIC MUSHROOM & BEEF SOUP (M)

MEDIUM

Serves: 6

Prep Time: 10 minutes

Cook Time: 40 minutes

Difficulty Level: 2

Cost: $$

Calories: 315
Carbs: 5g
Fiber: 1g
Net Carbs: 4g
Fat: 19g
Protein: 30g

Calories from:
Carbs: 5%
Fats: 56%
Protein: 39%

Ingredients:

- 1 pound beef chuck, cubed
- 1½ cups cremini mushrooms
- 6 cups beef broth
- ½ cup heavy cream
- ½ cup whipped cream cheese
- 1 yellow onion, chopped
- 2 cloves garlic, chopped
- Salt & pepper, to taste
- 1 tablespoon coconut oil, for cooking

Directions:

1. Add the coconut oil to a skillet and brown the beef.

2. Once cooked, add the beef to the base of a stockpot with all of the ingredients minus the heavy cream. Mix well.

3. Bring to a simmer and whisk again until the cream cheese is mixed evenly into the soup.

4. Cook for 30 minutes.

5. Warm the heavy cream, and then add to the soup.

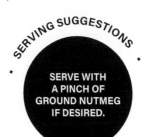

SERVING SUGGESTIONS

SERVE WITH A PINCH OF GROUND NUTMEG IF DESIRED.

CROCK-POT TURKEY TACO SOUP (H)

HIGH

Serves: 6

Prep Time: 10 minutes

Cook Time: 4 hours

Difficulty Level: 1

Cost: $

Calories: 335
Carbs: 6g
Fiber: 1g
Net Carbs: 5g
Fat: 23g
Protein: 28g

Calories from:
Carbs: 6%
Fats: 61%
Protein: 33%

Ingredients:

- 1 pound ground turkey
- 5 cups chicken bone broth (you can also use regular chicken broth)
- 1 cup canned diced tomatoes (no sugar added)
- 1 cup whipped cream cheese
- 1 yellow onion, chopped
- 1 tablespoon chili powder
- 1 teaspoon cumin
- 1 teaspoon garlic powder
- 1 teaspoon onion powder

Directions:

1. Add all the ingredients to the base of a Crock-Pot minus the cream cheese and cover with the chicken broth.

2. Set on high and cook for 4 hours adding in the cream cheese at the 3.5 hour mark.

3. Stir well before serving.

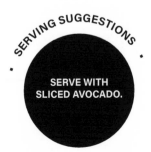

SERVING SUGGESTIONS

SERVE WITH SLICED AVOCADO.

SLOW COOKER LAMB & CAULIFLOWER SOUP (M)

MEDIUM

Serves: 6

Prep Time: 10 minutes

Cook Time: 4 hours

Difficulty Level: 1

Cost: $$

Calories: 263
Carbs: 6g
Fiber: 2g
Net Carbs: 4g
Fat: 14g
Protein: 27g

Calories from:
Carbs: 6%
Fats: 50%
Protein: 43%

Ingredients:

- 1 pound ground lamb
- 5 cups beef broth
- 1 cauliflower head, cut into florets
- 1 cup heavy cream
- 1 yellow onion, chopped
- 2 cloves garlic, chopped
- 1 tablespoon freshly chopped thyme
- ½ teaspoon cracked black pepper
- ½ teaspoon salt

Directions:

1. Add the ground lamb and cauliflower to the base of a stockpot.

2. Add in the remaining ingredients minus the heavy cream, and cook on high for 4 hours.

3. Warm the heavy cream before adding to the soup. Use an immersion blender to blend the soup until creamy.

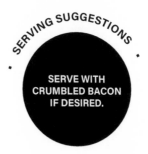

SERVING SUGGESTIONS

SERVE WITH CRUMBLED BACON IF DESIRED.

MEDIUM

Serves: 4

Prep Time: 10 minutes

Cook Time: 4 hours

Difficulty Level: 1

Cost: $$

Calories: 171
Carbs: 6g
Fiber: 1g
Net Carbs: 5g
Fat: 6g
Protein: 22g

Calories from:
Carbs: 12%
Fats: 33%
Protein: 54%

LEMON CHICKEN SOUP (M)

Ingredients:

- 2 boneless, skinless chicken breasts
- 6 cups chicken broth
- ¼ cup freshly squeezed lemon juice
- 2 tablespoons chives, chopped
- 1 yellow onion, chopped
- 2 cloves garlic, chopped
- Salt & pepper, to taste

Directions:

1. Add all the ingredients to a slow cooker and cook on high for 4 hours.

2. Once cooked, shred the chicken and stir back into the soup.

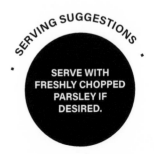

SERVING SUGGESTIONS

SERVE WITH FRESHLY CHOPPED PARSLEY IF DESIRED.

HAMBURGER & TOMATO SOUP (M)

MEDIUM

Serves: 6

Prep Time: 10 minutes

Cook Time: 4 hours

Difficulty Level: 1

Cost: $$

Calories: 209
Carbs: 5g
Fiber: 1g
Net Carbs: 4g
Fat: 9g
Protein: 26g

Calories from:
Carbs: 8%
Fats: 40%
Protein: 52%

Ingredients:

- 1 pound lean ground beef
- ½ cup no-sugar added marinara sauce
- ½ cup beef broth
- ½ cup shredded cheddar cheese
- 1 yellow onion, chopped
- 2 cloves garlic, chopped
- Salt & pepper, to taste

Directions:

1. Add all the ingredients to a slow cooker minus the shredded cheese and cook on high for 4 hours.

2. Stir in the cheese and serve.

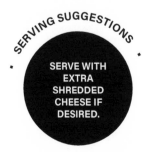

SERVING SUGGESTIONS

SERVE WITH EXTRA SHREDDED CHEESE IF DESIRED.

VEGETABLE BEEF SOUP (M)

MEDIUM

Serves: 6

Prep Time: 10 minutes

Cook Time: 4-6 hours

Difficulty Level: 1

Cost: $$

Calories: 185

Carbs: 5g

Fiber: 1g

Net Carbs: 4g

Fat: 6g

Protein: 7g

Calories from:
Carbs: 9%
Fats: 30%
Protein: 61%

Ingredients:

* 1 pound lean ground beef
* 4 cups beef broth
* 1 zucchini, diced
* 2 stalks celery, chopped
* ½ cup diced tomatoes
* 1 yellow onion, chopped
* 2 cloves garlic, chopped
* 1 teaspoon freshly chopped thyme
* 1 teaspoon freshly chopped rosemary
* Salt & pepper, to taste

Directions:

1. Add all the ingredients to a slow cooker and cook on high for 4 to 6 hours.

2. Stir well before serving.

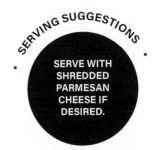

SERVING SUGGESTIONS

SERVE WITH SHREDDED PARMESAN CHEESE IF DESIRED.

LAMB TACO SOUP (M)

MEDIUM

Serves: 6

Prep Time: 10 minutes

Cook Time: 4-6 hours

Difficulty Level: 1

Cost: $$

Calories: 265
Carbs: 6g
Fiber: 1g
Net Carbs: 5g
Fat: 13g
Protein: 30g

Calories from:
Carbs: 8%
Fats: 46%
Protein: 47%

Ingredients:

- 1 pound ground lamb
- 4 cups beef broth
- 1 cup shredded cheddar cheese
- 1 cup diced tomatoes
- 1 green bell pepper, chopped
- 1 yellow onion, chopped
- 2 cloves garlic, chopped
- 1 teaspoon ground cumin
- 1 teaspoon ground coriander
- 1 teaspoon paprika
- ½ teaspoon cayenne pepper
- Salt & pepper, to taste

Directions:

1. Add all the ingredients to a slow cooker minus the shredded cheese and cook on high for 4 to 6 hours.

2. Stir in the shredded cheese and serve.

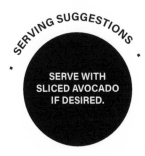

SERVING SUGGESTIONS

SERVE WITH SLICED AVOCADO IF DESIRED.

Vegetarian Soups

MEDIUM

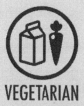

VEGETARIAN

Serves: 8

Prep Time: 15 minutes

Cook Time: 40 minutes

Difficulty Level: 2

Cost: $$

Calories: 73
Carbs: 7g
Fiber: 2g
Net Carbs: 5g
Fat: 3g
Protein: 4g

Calories from:
Carbs: 32%
Fats: 43%
Protein: 25%

CARROT, GINGER & TURMERIC SOUP (V)(M)

Ingredients:

- 6 cups vegetable broth
- ¼ cup full-fat unsweetened coconut milk
- ¾ pound carrots, peeled and chopped
- 2 teaspoons grated ginger
- 1 teaspoon ground turmeric
- 1 sweet yellow onion, chopped
- 2 cloves garlic, chopped
- Pinch of sea salt & pepper, to taste

Directions:

1. Add all the ingredients minus the coconut milk to a stockpot over medium heat and bring to a boil. Reduce to a simmer and cook for 40 minutes or until the carrots are tender.

2. Use an immersion blender and blend the soup until smooth. Stir in the coconut milk.

3. Enjoy right away and freeze any leftovers.

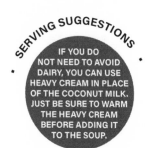

SERVING SUGGESTIONS

IF YOU DO NOT NEED TO AVOID DAIRY, YOU CAN USE HEAVY CREAM IN PLACE OF THE COCONUT MILK. JUST BE SURE TO WARM THE HEAVY CREAM BEFORE ADDING IT TO THE SOUP.

MEDIUM

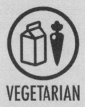

VEGETARIAN

Serves: 6

Prep Time: 15 minutes

Cook Time: 30 minutes

Difficulty Level: 2

Cost: $$

Calories: 104

Carbs: 6g

Fiber: 1g

Net Carbs: 5g

Fat: 7g

Protein: 6g

Calories from:
Carbs: 19%
Fats: 59%
Protein: 22%

VEGETARIAN GARLIC, TOMATO & ONION SOUP
(V)(M)

Ingredients:

- 6 cups vegetable broth
- ½ cup full-fat unsweetened coconut milk
- 1½ cups canned diced tomatoes
- 1 yellow onion, chopped
- 3 cloves garlic, chopped
- 1 teaspoon Italian seasoning
- 1 bay leaf
- Pinch of salt & pepper, to taste
- Fresh basil, for serving

Directions:

1. Add all the ingredients minus the coconut milk and fresh basil to a stockpot over medium heat and bring to a boil. Reduce to a simmer and cook for 30 minutes.

2. Remove the bay leaf, and then use an immersion blender to blend the soup until smooth. Stir in the coconut milk.

3. Garnish with fresh basil and serve.

SERVING SUGGESTIONS

IF YOU DO NOT NEED TO AVOID DAIRY, YOU CAN SERVE WITH FRESHLY GRATED PARMESAN CHEESE.

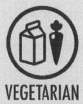

HIGH

VEGETARIAN

Serves: 6

Prep Time: 15 minutes

Cook Time: 30 minutes

Difficulty Level: 1

Cost: $$

Calories: 146

Carbs: 7g

Fiber: 2g

Net Carbs: 5g

Fat: 11g

Protein: 6g

Calories from:
Carbs: 14%
Fats: 69%
Protein: 17%

PUMPKIN, COCONUT & SAGE SOUP

(V)(H)

Ingredients:

- 6 cups vegetable broth
- 1 cup canned pumpkin
- 1 cup full-fat coconut milk
- 1 teaspoon freshly chopped sage
- 2 cloves garlic, chopped
- Pinch of salt & pepper, to taste

Directions:

1. Add all the ingredients minus the coconut milk to a stockpot over medium heat and bring to a boil. Reduce to a simmer and cook for 30 minutes.

2. Add the coconut milk and stir.

SERVING SUGGESTIONS

IF YOU DO NOT NEED TO AVOID DAIRY, YOU CAN USE HEAVY CREAM INSTEAD OF COCONUT MILK IF PREFERRED.

Creamy Soups

ITALIAN BEEF SOUP (M)

MEDIUM

Serves: 6

Prep Time: 10 minutes

Cook Time: 4 hours

Difficulty Level: 1

Cost: $$

Calories: 241

Carbs: 4g

Fiber: 1g

Net Carbs: 3g

Fat: 14g

Protein: 25g

Calories from:
Carbs: 5%
Fats: 53%
Protein: 42%

Ingredients:

- 1 pound lean ground beef
- 1 cup beef broth
- 1 cup heavy cream
- ½ cup shredded mozzarella cheese
- ½ cup diced tomatoes
- 1 yellow onion, chopped
- 2 cloves garlic, chopped
- 1 tablespoon Italian seasoning
- Salt & pepper, to taste

Directions:

1. Add all the ingredients to a slow cooker minus the heavy cream and mozzarella cheese. Cook on high for 4 hours.

2. Warm the heavy cream, and then add the warmed cream and cheese to the soup. Stir well and serve.

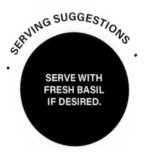

SERVING SUGGESTIONS

SERVE WITH FRESH BASIL IF DESIRED.

BACON & CHEESE SOUP (H)

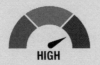

HIGH

Serves: 6

Prep Time: 15 minutes

Cook Time: 40 minutes

Difficulty Level: 2

Cost: $$

Calories: 498
Carbs: 5g
Fiber: 1g
Net Carbs: 4g
Fat: 34g
Protein: 41g

Calories from:
Carbs: 3%
Fats: 63%
Protein: 34%

Ingredients:

- 1 pound of lean ground beef
- 6 slices uncured bacon
- 6 cups beef broth
- 1 cup heavy cream
- 1 cup shredded cheddar cheese
- 1 yellow onion, chopped
- 1 teaspoon garlic powder
- ½ teaspoon onion powder
- ½ teaspoon cumin
- ½ teaspoon paprika
- ½ cup sour cream, for serving
- 1 tablespoon coconut oil, for cooking

Directions:

1. Add the coconut oil to a skillet and cook the bacon until crispy. Allow the bacon to cool and chop into small pieces. Set aside.

2. Once cooked, add the lean ground beef to the same skillet with the bacon fat and cook until browned.

3. Add the onions and cook for another 2 to 3 minutes.

4. Add all the ingredients minus the bacon, heavy cream, sour cream and cheese to a stockpot and stir. Cook for 25 minutes.

5. Warm the heavy cream, and then add the warmed cream and cheese and serve with the bacon and a dollop of sour cream.

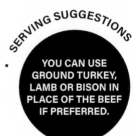

SERVING SUGGESTIONS

YOU CAN USE GROUND TURKEY, LAMB OR BISON IN PLACE OF THE BEEF IF PREFERRED.

CHEESY CHICKEN SOUP (M)

MEDIUM

Serves: 6

Prep Time: 20 minutes

Cook Time: 33-40 minutes

Difficulty Level: 2

Cost: $$

Calories: 157
Carbs: 5g
Fiber: 1g
Net Carbs: 4g
Fat: 7g
Protein: 17g

Calories from:
Carbs: 11%
Fats: 43%
Protein: 46%

Ingredients:

- 2 boneless, skinless chicken breasts
- 2 cups chicken broth
- 2 cups water
- 1 cup whipped cream cheese
- ½ cup shredded cheddar cheese
- 1 yellow onion, chopped
- 2 cloves garlic, chopped
- 1 teaspoon chili powder
- ½ teaspoon cumin
- ½ teaspoon salt
- ¼ teaspoon black pepper
- 1 tablespoon coconut oil, for cooking

Directions:

1. Heat a large skillet over medium heat with a ½ tablespoon of the coconut oil.

2. Brown the chicken breasts until cooked through. Set aside.

3. Add the garlic and onion to a large stockpot with the remaining 1 tablespoon of the coconut oil and sauté until translucent over low to medium heat. This should take about 3 to 5 minutes.

continue in the next page ▶

SERVING SUGGESTIONS

GARNISH WITH GREEN ONIONS IF DESIRED.

CHEESY CHICKEN SOUP (M)

MEDIUM

Serves: 6

Prep Time: 20 minutes

Cook Time: 33-40 minutes

Difficulty Level: 2

Cost: $$

Calories: 157
Carbs: 5g
Fiber: 1g
Net Carbs: 4g
Fat: 7g
Protein: 17g

Calories from:
Carbs: 11%
Fats: 43%
Protein: 46%

4. Add this chicken broth and water.

5. Whisk in the cream cheese and keep whisking over low to medium heat until combined.

6. Add in the spices and bring to a boil.

7. While the water is boiling, cut the chicken into bite-sized pieces and add to the stockpot.

8. Reduce to a simmer and cook for 30 to 35 minutes.

9. Stir in the cheddar cheese and serve.

GARLICKY CHICKEN SOUP (M)

MEDIUM

Serves: 6

Prep Time: 10 minutes

Cook Time: 15 minutes

Difficulty Level: 1

Cost: $

Calories: 128
Carbs: 2g
Fiber: 0g
Net Carbs: 2g
Fat: 6g
Protein: 16g

Calories from:
Carbs: 6%
Fats: 43%
Protein: 51%

Ingredients:

- 2 boneless, skinless chicken breasts
- 4 cups chicken broth
- ½ cup whipped cream cheese
- 3 cloves garlic, chopped
- 1 teaspoon thyme
- 1 teaspoon salt
- ¼ teaspoon black pepper
- 1 tablespoon butter for cooking

Directions:

1. Preheat a stockpot over medium heat with the butter.

2. Add the chicken and brown until completely cooked through. Remove from heat.

3. Shred the chicken and add it back to the stockpot along with the remaining ingredients minus the cream cheese.

4. Bring to a simmer.

5. Add in the cream cheese and whisk until there are no more clumps.

6. Simmer for 10 minutes and serve.

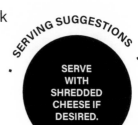

SERVING SUGGESTIONS

SERVE WITH SHREDDED CHEESE IF DESIRED.

BROCCOLI CHEDDAR & BACON SOUP (H)

HIGH

Serves: 6

Prep Time: 10 minutes

Cook Time: 10 minutes

Difficulty Level: 1

Cost: $

Calories: 220

Carbs: 4g

Fiber: 1g

Net Carbs: 3g

Fat: 18g

Protein: 11g

Calories from:
Carbs: 6%
Fats: 74%
Protein: 20%

Ingredients:

- 2 cups chicken broth
- 1 cup broccoli florets finely chopped
- 1 cup heavy cream
- 1 cup shredded cheddar cheese
- ½ white onion, chopped
- 2 cloves garlic, chopped
- 3 slices cooked bacon, crumbled for serving
- ½ teaspoon salt
- ¼ teaspoon black pepper

Directions:

1. Add all the ingredients minus the heavy cream, cheddar cheese and bacon to a stockpot over medium heat.

2. Bring to a simmer and cook for 5 minutes.

3. Warm the cream, and then add the warm cream and cheddar cheese. Whisk until smooth.

4. Serve with crumbled bacon.

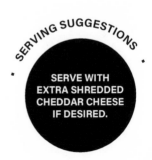

SERVING SUGGESTIONS

SERVE WITH EXTRA SHREDDED CHEDDAR CHEESE IF DESIRED.

TOMATO BISQUE SOUP (H)

HIGH

Serves: 6

Prep Time: 10 minutes

Cook Time: 40 minutes

Difficulty Level: 1

Cost: $

Calories: 144

Carbs: 4g

Fiber: 1g

Net Carbs: 3g

Fat: 12g

Protein: 4g

Calories from:
Carbs: 9%
Fats: 79%
Protein: 12%

Ingredients:

* 3 cups canned whole, peeled tomatoes
* 4 cups chicken broth
* 1 cup heavy cream
* 3 cloves garlic, chopped
* 2 tablespoons butter
* 1 teaspoon freshly chopped thyme
* Salt & black pepper, to taste

Directions:

1. Add the butter to the bottom of a stockpot.

2. Add in all the remaining ingredients minus the heavy cream. Bring to a boil, and then simmer for 40 minutes.

3. Warm the heavy cream, and then stir into the soup.

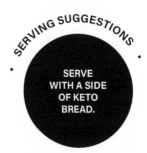

SERVING SUGGESTIONS

SERVE WITH A SIDE OF KETO BREAD.

CREAMY TURKEY SOUP (H)

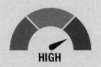

HIGH

Serves: 7

Prep Time: 15 minutes

Cook Time: 4 hours

Difficulty Level: 1

Cost: $$

Calories: 216
Carbs: 6g
Fiber: 1g
Net Carbs: 5g
Fat: 14g
Protein: 17g

Calories from:
Carbs: 9%
Fats: 59%
Protein: 32%

Ingredients:

- 1 pound turkey breast, cubed
- 5 cups chicken broth
- 1 cup cream cheese
- 1 carrot, chopped
- 1 stalk celery, chopped
- 3 cloves garlic, chopped
- 1 teaspoon freshly chopped rosemary
- Salt & black pepper, to taste

Directions:

1. Add all the ingredients minus the cream cheese to the base of a slow cooker.

2. Cook on high for 4 hours.

3. Stir in the cream cheese until well combined.

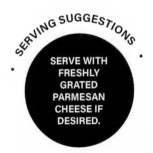

SERVING SUGGESTIONS

SERVE WITH FRESHLY GRATED PARMESAN CHEESE IF DESIRED.

CARROT GINGER SOUP (H)

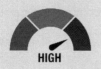

HIGH

Serves: 6

Prep Time: 15 minutes

Cook Time: 4 hours

Difficulty Level: 1

Cost: $$

Calories: 135
Carbs: 9g
Fiber: 2g
Net Carbs: 7g
Fat: 9g
Protein: 5g

Calories from:
Carbs: 22%
Fats: 63%
Protein: 16%

Ingredients:

- 1 cup heavy cream
- 5 cups chicken broth
- 6 carrots, chopped
- 2 tablespoons freshly chopped ginger
- 3 cloves garlic, chopped
- 1 teaspoon freshly chopped rosemary
- Salt & black pepper, to taste

Directions:

1. Add all the ingredients minus the heavy cream to the base of a slow cooker.

2. Cook on high for 4 hours.

3. Warm the heavy cream, and then add to the soup.

4. Use an immersion blender and blend until smooth.

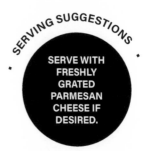

SERVING SUGGESTIONS

SERVE WITH FRESHLY GRATED PARMESAN CHEESE IF DESIRED.

CINNAMON HARVEST BUTTERNUT SQUASH SOUP (H)

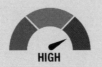

HIGH

Serves: 8

Prep Time: 15 minutes

Cook Time: 4-6 hours

Difficulty Level: 1

Cost: $$

Calories: 95
Carbs: 6g
Fiber: 1g
Net Carbs: 5g
Fat: 7g
Protein: 4g

Calories from:
Carbs: 20%
Fats: 64%
Protein: 16%

Ingredients:

- 1½ cups butternut squash, cubed
- 1 cup heavy cream
- 5 cups chicken broth
- 1 carrot, chopped
- 3 cloves garlic, chopped
- 2 teaspoons ground cinnamon
- ½ teaspoon ground nutmeg
- ½ teaspoon ground cloves
- Salt & black pepper, to taste

Directions:

1. Add all the ingredients minus the heavy cream to the base of a slow cooker.

2. Cook on high for 4 to 6 hours.

3. Warm the heavy cream, and then add to the soup.

4. Use an immersion blender and blend until smooth.

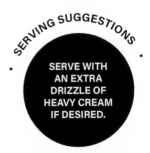

SERVING SUGGESTIONS

SERVE WITH AN EXTRA DRIZZLE OF HEAVY CREAM IF DESIRED.

44

PUMPKIN NUTMEG SOUP (H)

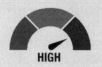

HIGH

Serves: 8

Prep Time: 15 minutes

Cook Time: 4-6 hours

Difficulty Level: 1

Cost: $$

Calories: 96
Carbs: 6g
Fiber: 2g
Net Carbs: 4g
Fat: 7g
Protein: 4g

Calories from:
Carbs: 17%
Fats: 66%
Protein: 17%

Ingredients:

- 1½ cups pumpkin, cubed
- 1 cup heavy cream
- 5 cups chicken broth
- 3 cloves garlic, chopped
- 2 teaspoons ground cinnamon
- ½ teaspoon ground nutmeg
- ½ teaspoon ground cloves
- Salt & black pepper, to taste

Directions:

1. Add all the ingredients minus the heavy cream to the base of a slow cooker.

2. Cook on high for 4 to 6 hours.

3. Warm the heavy cream, and then add to the soup.

4. Use an immersion blender and blend until smooth.

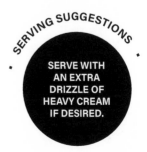

SERVING SUGGESTIONS

SERVE WITH AN EXTRA DRIZZLE OF HEAVY CREAM IF DESIRED.

CREAM OF SPINACH MOZZARELLA SOUP (H)

HIGH

Serves: 4

Prep Time: 10 minutes

Cook Time: 15 minutes

Difficulty Level: 1

Cost: $$

Calories: 151
Carbs: 3g
Fiber: 0g
Net Carbs: 3g
Fat: 13g
Protein: 6g

Calories from:
Carbs: 8%
Fats: 76%
Protein: 16%

Ingredients:

- 2 cups chicken broth
- 1 cup heavy cream
- 1 cup shredded mozzarella cheese
- 1 cup fresh spinach, chopped
- 3 cloves garlic, chopped
- 1 teaspoon onion powder
- 1 teaspoon dried thyme
- Salt & black pepper, to taste

Directions:

1. Add all the ingredients minus the heavy cream and mozzarella to the base of a stockpot.

2. Bring to a boil, and then simmer for 10 minutes.

3. Warm the heavy cream, and then add to the soup along with mozzarella. Stir until the cheese has melted.

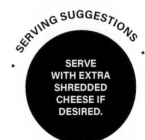

SERVING SUGGESTIONS

SERVE WITH EXTRA SHREDDED CHEESE IF DESIRED.

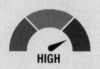

HIGH

Serves: 4

Prep Time: 10 minutes

Cook Time: 15 minutes

Difficulty Level: 1

Cost: $$

Calories: 228
Carbs: 7g
Fiber: 2g
Net Carbs: 5g
Fat: 17g
Protein: 12g

Calories from:
Carbs: 9%
Fats: 69%
Protein: 22%

CREAM OF ASPARAGUS & PARMESAN SOUP (H)

Ingredients:

- 2 cups chicken broth
- 1 cup heavy cream
- 1 cup shredded Parmesan cheese
- 1 cup asparagus finely chopped
- 1 yellow onion, chopped
- 3 cloves garlic, chopped
- 1 teaspoon dried thyme
- Salt & black pepper, to taste

Directions:

1. Add all the ingredients minus the heavy cream and Parmesan cheese to the base of a stockpot.

2. Bring to a boil, and then simmer for 10 minutes.

3. Warm the heavy cream, and then add to the soup along with the Parmesan cheese. Stir until the cheese has melted and serve.

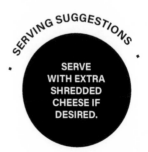

SERVING SUGGESTIONS

SERVE WITH EXTRA SHREDDED CHEESE IF DESIRED.

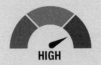

HIGH

MOZZARELLA TOMATO & BASIL SOUP (H)

Serves: 6

Prep Time: 15 minutes

Cook Time: 30 minutes

Difficulty Level: 2

Cost: $$

Calories: 122
Carbs: 5g
Fiber: 1g
Net Carbs: 4g
Fat: 9g
Protein: 6g

Calories from:
Carbs: 13%
Fats: 67%
Protein: 20%

Ingredients:

- 4 cups vegetable broth
- 1 cup heavy cream
- 1 cup canned diced tomatoes
- 1 yellow onion, chopped
- 2 cloves garlic, chopped
- 1 cup shredded mozzarella cheese
- Freshly chopped basil, for serving

Directions:

1. Add all of the ingredients minus the heavy cream, cheese and fresh basil to a stockpot over medium heat. Bring to a boil, and then reduce to a simmer.

2. Simmer for 30 minutes.

3. While the soup is cooking, warm the heavy cream over low heat and add to the soup once cooked.

4. Use an immersion blender and blend until smooth.

5. Stir in the mozzarella cheese and top with fresh basil.

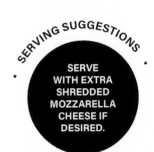

SERVING SUGGESTIONS

SERVE WITH EXTRA SHREDDED MOZZARELLA CHEESE IF DESIRED.

48

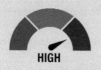

HIGH

Serves: 8

Prep Time: 10 minutes

Cook Time: 60 minutes

Difficulty Level: 1

Cost: $$

Calories: 225

Carbs: 8g

Fiber: 3g

Net Carbs: 5g

Fat: 21g

Protein: 4g

Calories from:
Carbs: 9%
Fats: 84%
Protein: 7%

CREAM OF MACADAMIA SOUP (H)

Ingredients:

- 4 carrots, peeled chopped
- 1 leek (white portion only)
- 2 garlic cloves, peeled
- 1 cup macadamia nuts, finely chopped or ground
- 4 tablespoons butter
- 4 cups chicken broth
- ¼ cup heavy cream
- 2 tablespoons chopped fresh cilantro (reserve 1 tablespoon for garnish)
- 1 teaspoon turmeric
- 1 teaspoon salt
- ½ teaspoon black pepper

Directions:

1. Add all of the ingredients, starting with the butter, to a large stockpot. Bring to a boil, and then reduce heat and simmer for 1 hour.

2. Use an immersion blender and blend until smooth.

3. Garnish with fresh cilantro, if desired.

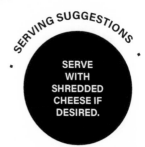

SERVING SUGGESTIONS

SERVE WITH SHREDDED CHEESE IF DESIRED.

Spicy Soups

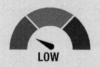

LOW

Serves: 6

Prep Time: 10 minutes

Cook Time: 4 hours

Difficulty Level: 1

Cost: $

Calories: 108

Carbs: 4g

Fiber: 1g

Net Carbs: 3g

Fat: 3g

Protein: 16g

Calories from:
Carbs: 12%
Fats: 26%
Protein: 62%

SPICY LIME CILANTRO SOUP (L)

Ingredients:

- 6 cups chicken broth
- 3 boneless, skinless chicken breasts
- Juice from 1 lime
- 1 yellow onion, chopped
- 2 cloves garlic, chopped
- 1 jalapeno pepper, seeded and sliced
- 1 handful fresh cilantro
- Salt & black pepper, to taste

Directions:

1. Add all the ingredients minus the cilantro, salt and black pepper to the base of a slow cooker and cook on high for 4 hours.

2. Add the cilantro and season with salt and black pepper.

3. Shred the chicken and serve.

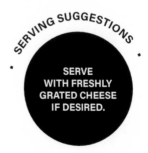

SERVING SUGGESTIONS

SERVE WITH FRESHLY GRATED CHEESE IF DESIRED.

ZESTY LEMON CHICKEN SOUP (L)

LOW

Serves: 6

Prep Time: 10 minutes

Cook Time: 4 hours

Difficulty Level: 1

Cost: $

Calories: 108
Carbs: 4g
Fiber: 1g
Net Carbs: 3g
Fat: 3g
Protein: 16g

Calories from:
Carbs: 12%
Fats: 26%
Protein: 62%

Ingredients:

- 6 cups chicken broth
- 3 boneless, skinless chicken breasts
- Juice from 1 lemon
- 1 yellow onion, chopped
- 2 cloves garlic, chopped
- 1 teaspoon cayenne pepper
- 1 teaspoon dried thyme
- 1 handful of fresh parsley, minced
- Salt & black pepper, to taste

Directions:

1. Add all the ingredients minus the salt, black pepper and parsley to the base of a slow cooker minus the parsley and cook on high for 4 hours.

2. Add the parsley and season with salt and black pepper.

3. Shred the chicken and serve.

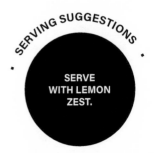

SERVING SUGGESTIONS

SERVE WITH LEMON ZEST.

SPICY ITALIAN SOUP (M)

MEDIUM

Serves: 6

Prep Time: 10 minutes

Cook Time: 4 hours

Difficulty Level: 1

Cost: $

Calories: 125

Carbs: 5g

Fiber: 1g

Net Carbs: 4g

Fat: 4g

Protein: 17g

Calories from:
Carbs: 13%
Fats: 30%
Protein: 57%

Ingredients:

- 6 cups chicken broth
- 3 boneless, skinless chicken breasts
- 1 cup canned diced tomatoes
- 1 yellow onion, chopped
- 2 cloves garlic, chopped
- 1 cup shredded mozzarella cheese
- 1 jalapeno pepper, seeded and sliced
- 1 teaspoon dried thyme
- 1 teaspoon dried oregano
- Salt & black pepper, to taste

Directions:

1. Add all the ingredients minus the salt and black pepper to the base of a slow cooker minus the cheese and cook on high for 4 hours.

2. Stir in the cheese and season with salt and black pepper.

3. Shred the chicken and serve.

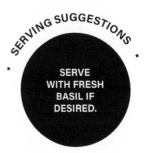

SERVING SUGGESTIONS

SERVE WITH FRESH BASIL IF DESIRED.

JALAPENO & LIME SHRIMP SOUP (M)

MEDIUM

Serves: 6

Prep Time: 10 minutes

Cook Time: 35 minutes

Difficulty Level: 1

Cost: $$

Calories: 153
Carbs: 6g
Fiber: 1g
Net Carbs: 5g
Fat: 5g
Protein: 21g

Calories from:
Carbs: 13%
Fats: 30%
Protein: 56%

Ingredients:

* 4 cups chicken broth
* Juice from 1 lime
* 1 pound peeled, deveined shrimp
* 1 yellow onion, chopped
* 1 shallot, chopped
* 3 cloves garlic, chopped
* 1 jalapeno pepper, seeded and sliced
* Salt & black pepper, to taste
* 1 tablespoon coconut oil for cooking

Directions:

1. Add the coconut oil to a large stockpot over medium heat.

2. Add the shrimp, onion, shallot and garlic and cook until the shrimp are cooked through and pink.

3. Add the remaining ingredients minus the salt and black pepper, and bring to a boil.

4. Reduce the heat to a simmer and cook for 30 minutes.

5. Season with salt and black pepper and serve.

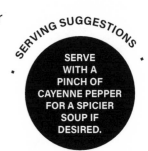

SERVING SUGGESTIONS

SERVE WITH A PINCH OF CAYENNE PEPPER FOR A SPICIER SOUP IF DESIRED.

Cold Soups

HIGH

VEGETARIAN

REFRESHING CREAMY MINT SOUP (V)(H)

Serves: 4

Prep Time: 10 minutes + 1 hour chilling time

Cook Time: None

Difficulty Level: 1

Cost: $$

Calories: 248

Carbs: 9g

Fiber: 5g

Net Carbs: 4g

Fat: 24g

Protein: 3g

Calories from:
Carbs: 7%
Fats: 89%
Protein: 5%

Ingredients:

- 1 ripe avocado
- ½ cucumber, sliced
- 1 cup full-fat unsweetened coconut milk
- 1 tablespoon freshly chopped mint leaves
- 1 tablespoon freshly squeezed lemon juice
- Pinch of salt

Directions:

1. Add all the ingredients to a high-speed blender and blend until creamy.

2. Chill in the refrigerator for 1 hour before serving.

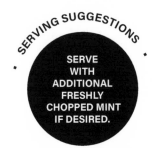

SERVING SUGGESTIONS

SERVE WITH ADDITIONAL FRESHLY CHOPPED MINT IF DESIRED.

HIGH

Serves: 4

Prep Time: 10 minutes +
1 hour chilling time

Cook Time: None

Difficulty Level: 1

Cost: $$

Calories: 289

Carbs: 10g

Fiber: 7g

Net Carbs: 3g

Fat: 26g

Protein: 6g

Calories from:
Carbs: 4%
Fats: 87%
Protein: 9%

GUACAMOLE SOUP (H)

Ingredients:

- 3 cups chicken broth
- ½ cup heavy cream
- 2 ripe avocados pitted
- ½ cup freshly chopped cilantro
- 1 tomato, chopped
- Salt & black pepper, to taste

Directions:

1. Add all the ingredients to a high-speed blender and blend until creamy.

2. Chill in the refrigerator for 1 hour before serving.

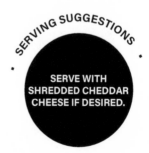

SERVING SUGGESTIONS

SERVE WITH
SHREDDED CHEDDAR
CHEESE IF DESIRED.

HIGH

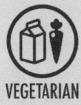

VEGETARIAN

Serves: 6

Prep Time: 10 minutes +
1 hour chilling time

Cook Time: None

Difficulty Level: 1

Cost: $$

Calories: 233

Carbs: 6g

Fiber: 1g

Net Carbs: 5g

Fat: 23g

Protein: 3g

Calories from:
Carbs: 8%
Fats: 87%
Protein: 5%

HERBED CREAM SOUP (V)(H)

Ingredients:

- 2 cups heavy cream
- 1 cup sour cream
- 1 cucumber, diced
- 1 tablespoon spicy brown mustard
- 1 tablespoon horseradish
- 2 tablespoons freshly chopped parsley
- 2 tablespoons freshly chopped dill
- 2 tablespoons freshly chopped mint
- Salt & black pepper, to taste

Directions:

1. Add all the ingredients to a large mixing bowl minus the cucumber. Use an immersion blender and blend until smooth.

2. Stir in the cucumber, and chill in the refrigerator for at least 1 hour before serving.

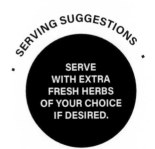

SERVING SUGGESTIONS

SERVE WITH EXTRA FRESH HERBS OF YOUR CHOICE IF DESIRED.

MEDIUM

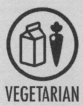

VEGETARIAN

Serves: 8

Prep Time: 15 minutes + 2 hour chilling time

Cook Time: None

Difficulty Level: 1

Cost: $$

Calories: 101

Carbs: 6g

Fiber: 0g

Net Carbs: 6g

Fat: 5g

Protein: 11g

Calories from:
Carbs: 21%
Fats: 40%
Protein: 39%

YOGURT & DILL SOUP (V)(M)

Ingredients:

- 4 cups full-fat, unsweetened Greek yogurt
- 2 cups very cold water (it's best to refrigerate the water a few hours before making the soup)
- 2 cloves garlic, chopped
- ¼ cup freshly chopped parsley
- ¼ cup freshly chopped dill
- 2 tablespoons freshly chopped mint
- Salt & black pepper, to taste

Directions:

1. Add all the ingredients to a large mixing bowl. Use an immersion blender and blend until smooth.

2. Chill for 2 hours in the refrigerator before serving.

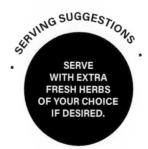

SERVING SUGGESTIONS

SERVE WITH EXTRA FRESH HERBS OF YOUR CHOICE IF DESIRED.

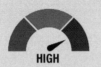

HIGH

ROSEMARY & THYME CUCUMBER SOUP (H)

Serves: 6

Prep Time: 15 minutes + 1 hour chilling time

Cook Time: None

Difficulty Level: 1

Cost: $$

Calories: 111

Carbs: 5g

Fiber: 1g

Net Carbs: 4g

Fat: 9g

Protein: 4g

Calories from:
Carbs: 14%
Fats: 72%
Protein: 14%

Ingredients:

- 4 cups chicken broth
- 1 cup heavy cream
- 2 cucumbers, sliced
- 1 teaspoon freshly chopped rosemary
- 1 teaspoon freshly chopped thyme
- 1 pinch of salt & black pepper, to taste

Directions:

1. Add all the ingredients to a large mixing bowl and whisk well.

2. Use an immersion blender and blend until smooth.

3. Chill for 1 hour before serving.

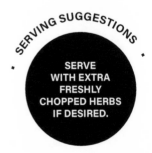

SERVING SUGGESTIONS

SERVE WITH EXTRA FRESHLY CHOPPED HERBS IF DESIRED.

MEDIUM

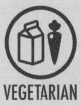

VEGETARIAN

Serves: 6

Prep Time: 15 minutes + 1 hour chilling time

Cook Time: None

Difficulty Level: 1

Cost: $$

Calories: 232

Carbs: 7g

Fiber: 5g

Net Carbs: 2g

Fat: 21g

Protein: 5g

Calories from:
Carbs: 4%
Fats: 87%
Protein: 9%

CREAMY CILANTRO & LIME SOUP (V)(H)

Ingredients:

- 4 cups vegetable broth
- 1 cup heavy cream
- 2 ripe avocados, pitted and sliced
- ½ cup freshly chopped cilantro
- 2 tablespoons freshly squeezed lime juice
- ½ teaspoon sea salt

Directions:

1. Add all the ingredients to a large mixing bowl and whisk well.

2. Use an immersion blender and blend until smooth.

3. Chill for 1 hour before serving.

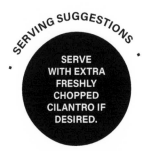

SERVING SUGGESTIONS

SERVE WITH EXTRA FRESHLY CHOPPED CILANTRO IF DESIRED.

Quick & Easy Soups -5 Ingredients or Less

HIGH

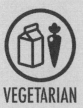

VEGETARIAN

Serves: 4

Prep Time: 15 minutes

Cook Time: 30 minutes

Difficulty Level: 1

Cost: $$

Calories: 158
Carbs: 5g
Fiber: 1g
Net Carbs: 4g
Fat: 13g
Protein: 7g

Calories from:
Carbs: 10%
Fats: 73%
Protein: 17%

QUICK CREAM OF ASPARAGUS SOUP (V)(H)

Ingredients:

- 4 cups vegetable broth
- 1 cup heavy cream
- 1 bunch asparagus, chopped into 1-inch pieces
- 2 cloves garlic, chopped
- 1 pinch of sea salt

Directions:

1. Add all the ingredients to a stockpot over medium heat minus the heavy cream and bring to a boil. Reduce to a simmer and cook for 30 minutes.

2. Warm the heavy cream, and then stir into the soup.

3. Use an immersion blender and blend until smooth.

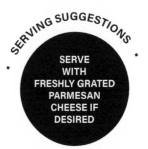

SERVING SUGGESTIONS

SERVE WITH FRESHLY GRATED PARMESAN CHEESE IF DESIRED

CREAM CHEESE & CHIVES CHICKEN NOODLE SOUP (H)

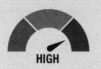

HIGH

Serves: 8

Prep Time: 15 minutes

Cook Time: 120 minutes-6 hours

Difficulty Level: 1

Cost: $$

Calories: 602

Carbs: 2g

Fiber: 0g

Net Carbs: 2g

Fat: 45g

Protein: 46g

Calories from:
Carbs: 1%
Fats: 68%
Protein: 31%

Ingredients:

* 6 cups chicken broth
* 1 cup heavy cream
* 1 cup whipped cream cheese
* 1 whole chicken
* 2 tablespoons freshly chopped chives
* Salt & black pepper, to taste

Directions:

1. Add the whole chicken to the base of a Crock-Pot or Instant Pot.

2. Add the chicken broth.

3. If using an Instant Pot, close the valve to sealing and set to 120 minutes on the manual setting. If using a Crock-Pot, cook on low for 6 hours.

4. Once cooked, remove the chicken and shred. Add the meat back to the soup and stir.

5. Warm the heavy cream, and then add the cream cheese and heavy cream and stir until combined.

6. Serve with fresh chives, season with salt and black pepper and serve.

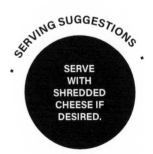

SERVING SUGGESTIONS

SERVE WITH SHREDDED CHEESE IF DESIRED.

SPICY SAUSAGE SOUP (M)

MEDIUM

Serves: 4

Prep Time: 10 minutes

Cook Time: 40 minutes

Difficulty Level: 1

Cost: $$

Calories: 107

Carbs: 6g

Fiber: 1g

Net Carbs: 5g

Fat: 6g

Protein: 8g

Calories from:
Carbs: 19%
Fats: 51%
Protein: 30%

Ingredients:

- 4 cups chicken broth
- 4 sausage links, sliced
- 1 cup cauliflower florets
- 1 yellow onion, chopped
- 1 teaspoon paprika
- Sea salt & pepper, to taste

Directions:

1. Add all the ingredients minus the salt and black pepper to a stockpot over medium heat and bring to a boil. Reduce to a simmer and cook for 40 minutes.

2. Season with salt and black pepper and serve.

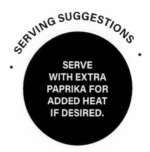

SERVING SUGGESTIONS

SERVE WITH EXTRA PAPRIKA FOR ADDED HEAT IF DESIRED.

MEDIUM

Serves: 6

Prep Time: 10 minutes

Cook Time: None

Difficulty Level: 1

Cost: $$

Calories: 270

Carbs: 6g

Fiber: 2g

Net Carbs: 4g

Fat: 14g

Protein: 29g

Calories from:
Carbs: 6%
Fats: 49%
Protein: 45%

VEGGIE BEEF SOUP (M)

Ingredients:

- 6 cups beef broth
- 1 cup heavy cream
- 1 pound lean ground beef
- 1 cup frozen mixed vegetables
- 1 yellow onion, chopped
- Salt & black pepper, to taste

Directions:

1. Add all the ingredients minus the salt, black pepper and heavy cream and bring to a boil. Reduce the heat to a simmer and cook for 40 minutes.

2. Before the soup is done cooking, warm the heavy cream, and then add once the soup is cooked.

3. Season with salt and black pepper and serve.

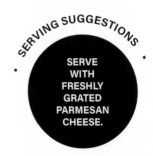

SERVING SUGGESTIONS

SERVE WITH FRESHLY GRATED PARMESAN CHEESE.

HIGH

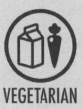

VEGETARIAN

Serves: 6

Prep Time: 10 minutes

Cook Time: 40 minutes

Difficulty Level: 1

Cost: $$

Calories: 129

Carbs: 6g

Fiber: 2g

Net Carbs: 4g

Fat: 9g

Protein: 7g

Calories from:
Carbs: 13%
Fats: 65%
Protein: 22%

CAULIFLOWER GARLIC SOUP (V)(H)

Ingredients:

- 6 cups vegetable broth
- 1 cup heavy cream
- 1 cauliflower head, cut into florets
- 4 cloves garlic, chopped
- 1 yellow onion, chopped
- Salt & black pepper, to taste

Directions:

1. Add all the ingredients minus the heavy cream, salt and black pepper to a stockpot and bring to a boil. Reduce heat to a simmer and cook for 40 minutes.

2. Warm the heavy cream, and then add to the soup.

3. Use an immersion blender and blend until smooth, season with salt and black pepper and serve.

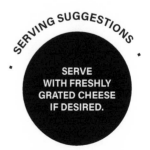

SERVING SUGGESTIONS

SERVE WITH FRESHLY GRATED CHEESE IF DESIRED.

CREAMY BROCCOLI & BACON SOUP (H)

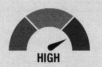

HIGH

Serves: 6

Prep Time: 10 minutes

Cook Time: 40 minutes

Difficulty Level: 1

Cost: $$

Calories: 175

Carbs: 4g

Fiber: 1g

Net Carbs: 3g

Fat: 14g

Protein: 9g

Calories from:
Carbs: 7%
Fats: 72%
Protein: 21%

Ingredients:

- 4 cups chicken broth
- 1 cup heavy cream
- 1 broccoli head, cut into florets
- 2 cloves garlic, chopped
- 4 slices bacon, chopped
- Salt & black pepper, to taste

Directions:

1. Add all the ingredients minus the heavy cream to a stockpot and bring to a boil. Reduce heat to a simmer and cook for 40 minutes.

2. Warm the heavy cream, and then add to the soup.

3. Season with salt and black pepper and serve.

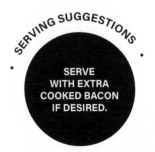

SERVING SUGGESTIONS

SERVE WITH EXTRA COOKED BACON IF DESIRED.

MEDIUM

Serves: 6

Prep Time: 10 minutes

Cook Time: 40 minutes

Difficulty Level: 1

Cost: $$

Calories: 215

Carbs: 4g

Fiber: 1g

Net Carbs: 3g

Fat: 11g

Protein: 27g

Calories from:
Carbs: 5%
Fats: 45%
Protein: 49%

TURKEY, SAUSAGE & KALE SOUP (M)

Ingredients:

- 6 cups chicken broth
- 1 pound ground turkey
- 2 turkey sausage links, sliced
- 1 cup kale, chopped
- 1 yellow onion, chopped
- Salt & black pepper, to taste

Directions:

1. Add all the ingredients minus the salt and black pepper to a stockpot and bring to a boil. Reduce heat to a simmer and cook for 40 minutes.

2. Season with salt and black pepper and serve.

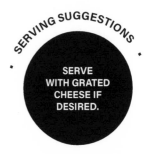

SERVING SUGGESTIONS

SERVE WITH GRATED CHEESE IF DESIRED.

Vegetarian Comfort Stews

LOW

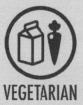

VEGETARIAN

Serves: 6

Prep Time: 10 minutes

Cook Time: 40 minutes

Difficulty Level: 1

Cost: $$

Calories: 62

Carbs: 9g

Fiber: 2g

Net Carbs: 7g

Fat: 1g

Protein: 4g

Calories from:
Carbs: 53%
Fats: 17%
Protein: 30%

PUMPKIN KALE VEGETARIAN STEW (V)(L)

Ingredients:

- 4 cups vegetable broth
- 1 cup pumpkin, cubed
- 2 carrots, chopped
- 1 yellow onion, chopped
- 2 cloves garlic, chopped
- 1 cup kale, chopped
- Salt & black pepper, to taste

Directions:

1. Add all the ingredients minus the salt and black pepper to a stockpot and bring to a boil. Reduce heat to a simmer and cook for 40 minutes.

2. Season with salt and black pepper and serve.

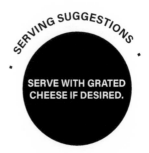

SERVING SUGGESTIONS

SERVE WITH GRATED CHEESE IF DESIRED.

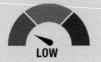

LOW

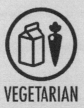

VEGETARIAN

Serves: 6

Prep Time: 10 minutes

Cook Time: 40 minutes

Difficulty Level: 1

Cost: $$

Calories: 61

Carbs: 8g

Fiber: 2g

Net Carbs: 6g

Fat: 1g

Protein: 5g

Calories from:
Carbs: 45%
Fats: 17%
Protein: 38%

NO BEAN CHILI (V)(L)

Ingredients:

- 4 cups vegetable broth
- 4 ounces tomato paste
- ¼ cup balsamic vinegar
- 1 yellow onion, chopped
- 1 green bell pepper, seeded and chopped

- 2 cloves garlic, chopped
- 2 teaspoons chili powder
- Salt & black pepper, to taste

Directions:

1. Add all the ingredients minus the salt and black pepper to a stockpot and bring to a boil. Reduce heat to a simmer and cook for 40 minutes.

2. Season with salt and black pepper and serve.

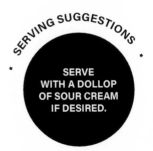

SERVING SUGGESTIONS

SERVE WITH A DOLLOP OF SOUR CREAM IF DESIRED.

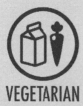

HIGH

VEGETARIAN

Serves: 6

Prep Time: 10 minutes

Cook Time: 40 minutes

Difficulty Level: 1

Cost: $

Calories: 142

Carbs: 8g

Fiber: 3g

Net Carbs: 5g

Fat: 11g

Protein: 5g

Calories from:
Carbs: 14%
Fats: 71%
Protein: 14%

ANTI-INFLAMMATORY TURMERIC STEW (V)(H)

Ingredients:

- 4 cups vegetable broth
- 1 cauliflower head, cut into florets
- 1 cup full-fat coconut milk
- 2 cloves garlic, chopped
- 1 yellow onion, chopped
- 2 teaspoons ground turmeric
- 1 teaspoon ground cinnamon
- 1 teaspoon dried oregano
- Salt & black pepper, to taste

Directions:

1. Add all the ingredients minus the salt, black pepper and coconut milk to a stockpot and bring to a boil. Reduce heat to a simmer and cook for 40 minutes.

2. Stir in the coconut milk.

3. Season with salt and black pepper and serve.

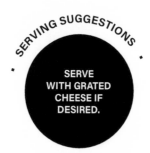

SERVING SUGGESTIONS

SERVE WITH GRATED CHEESE IF DESIRED.

HIGH

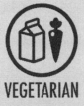

VEGETARIAN

Serves: 6

Prep Time: 10 minutes

Cook Time: 4 hours

Difficulty Level: 1

Cost: $

Calories: 157

Carbs: 9g

Fiber: 3g

Net Carbs: 6g

Fat: 11g

Protein: 7g

Calories from:
Carbs: 16%
Fats: 66%
Protein: 19%

HERBED BROCCOLI STEW (V)(H)

Ingredients:

- 6 cups vegetable broth
- 1 cup full-fat coconut milk
- 2 cups broccoli florets
- 1 cup canned diced tomatoes (no sugar added)
- 1 yellow onion, chopped
- 2 cloves garlic, chopped
- 1 teaspoon dried sage
- 1 teaspoon dried oregano
- 1 teaspoon dried rosemary
- Salt & black pepper, to taste

Directions:

1. Add all the ingredients minus the salt, black pepper and coconut milk to a slow cooker and cook on high for 4 hours.

2. Stir in the coconut milk and season with salt and black pepper.

SERVING SUGGESTIONS

SERVE WITH FRESHLY CHOPPED HERBS OF CHOICE IF DESIRED

HIGH

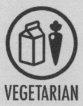

VEGETARIAN

Serves: 6

Prep Time: 15 minutes

Cook Time: 4 hours

Difficulty Level: 1

Cost: $$

Calories: 232
Carbs: 6g
Fiber: 1g
Net Carbs: 5g
Fat: 16g
Protein: 17g

Calories from:
Carbs: 9%
Fats: 62%
Protein: 29%

CREAMY MIXED VEGETABLE STEW (V)(H)

Ingredients:

- 4 cups vegetable broth
- 1 cup heavy cream
- 1 cup shredded Parmesan cheese
- 1 cup broccoli florets, chopped
- 1 cup canned diced tomatoes
- 1 yellow onion, chopped
- Salt & black pepper, to taste

Directions:

1. Add all the ingredients minus the heavy cream, salt and black pepper to the base of a slow cooker. Cook on high for 4 hours.

2. Once cooked, warm the cream, and then stir into the stew.

3. Season with salt and black pepper and serve.

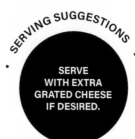

SERVING SUGGESTIONS

SERVE WITH EXTRA GRATED CHEESE IF DESIRED.

HIGH

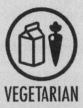

VEGETARIAN

Serves: 6

Prep Time: 10 minutes

Cook Time: 4 hours

Difficulty Level: 1

Cost: $$

Calories: 125

Carbs: 5g

Fiber: 1g

Net Carbs: 4g

Fat: 9g

Protein: 6g

Calories from:
Carbs: 13%
Fats: 67%
Protein: 20%

ASPARAGUS & MUSHROOM NUTMEG STEW (V)(H)

Ingredients:

- 6 cups vegetable broth
- 1 cup heavy cream
- 1 cup asparagus, chopped
- 1 cup cremini mushrooms
- 2 cloves garlic, chopped
- 1 yellow onion, chopped
- ½ teaspoon nutmeg
- Salt & black pepper, to taste

Directions:

1. Add all the ingredients minus the heavy cream, salt and black pepper to a slow cooker and cook on high for 4 hours.

2. Once cooked, warm the heavy cream, and then stir into the stew.

3. Season with salt and black pepper and serve.

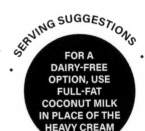

SERVING SUGGESTIONS

FOR A DAIRY-FREE OPTION, USE FULL-FAT COCONUT MILK IN PLACE OF THE HEAVY CREAM

76

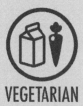

MEDIUM

VEGETARIAN

Serves: 4

Prep Time: 10 minutes

Cook Time: 20 minutes

Difficulty Level: 1

Cost: $

Calories: 141

Carbs: 8g

Fiber: 2g

Net Carbs: 6g

Fat: 8g

Protein: 11g

Calories from:
Carbs: 17%
Fats: 51%
Protein: 31%

BALSAMIC TOFU STEW (V)(M)

Ingredients:

- 2 cups vegetable broth
- ¼ cup balsamic vinegar
- 1½ cups firm tofu, cubed
- 1 green bell pepper, seeded and chopped
- 1 yellow onion, chopped
- 1 teaspoon garlic powder
- 1 tablespoon coconut oil, for cooking
- Salt & black pepper, to taste

Directions:

1. Add the coconut oil to a skillet over medium heat and sauté the tofu, bell pepper and onion for about 10 minutes.

2. Add the vegetable broth, balsamic and garlic powder and bring to a simmer. Cook for another 10 minutes or until the stew begins to thicken.

3. Season with salt and black pepper and serve.

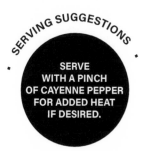

SERVING SUGGESTIONS

SERVE WITH A PINCH OF CAYENNE PEPPER FOR ADDED HEAT IF DESIRED.

Meat-Based Comfort Stews

BALSAMIC BEEF STEW (M)

MEDIUM

Serves: 6

Prep Time: 10 minutes

Cook Time: 6 hours

Difficulty Level: 1

Cost: $

Calories: 188

Carbs: 5g

Fiber: 1g

Net Carbs: 4g

Fat: 7g

Protein: 25g

Calories from:
Carbs: 9%
Fats: 35%
Protein: 56%

Ingredients:

- 1 pound sirloin steak, cubed
- 1 red onion, sliced
- 3 cloves garlic, chopped
- 2 carrots, chopped
- ¼ cup balsamic vinegar
- 1 cup beef broth
- ¼ cup parsley, freshly chopped
- 1 teaspoon salt
- ¼ teaspoon black pepper
- ¼ cup sour cream, for serving

Directions:

1. Add the sirloin steak to the base of a slow cooker and cook for 10 minutes.

2. Add in the remaining ingredients and cook on low for 6 hours.

3. Serve with a dollop of sour cream per serving.

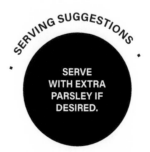

SERVING SUGGESTIONS

SERVE WITH EXTRA PARSLEY IF DESIRED.

MAC & CHEESE STEW (M)

MEDIUM

Serves: 6

Prep Time: 10 minutes

Cook Time: 4 hours

Difficulty Level: 1

Cost: $

Calories: 318

Carbs: 7g

Fiber: 1g

Net Carbs: 6g

Fat: 17g

Protein: 33g

Calories from:
Carbs: 8%
Fats: 50%
Protein: 43%

Ingredients:

- 1 pound lean ground beef
- 1 cup butternut squash, cubed
- 1 yellow onion, chopped
- 3 cloves garlic, chopped
- 2 cups shredded cheddar cheese
- 1 cup broccoli florets, chopped
- 1 teaspoon dried thyme
- Salt & black pepper, to taste

Directions:

1. Add all the ingredients minus the salt and black pepper to the base of a slow cooker and cook on high for 4 hours.

2. Season with salt and black pepper and serve.

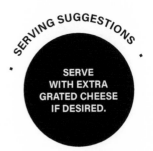

SERVING SUGGESTIONS

SERVE WITH EXTRA GRATED CHEESE IF DESIRED.

80

TURKEY, ONION & SAGE STEW (M)

MEDIUM

Serves: 6

Prep Time: 10 minutes

Cook Time: 4 hours

Difficulty Level: 1

Cost: $

Calories: 189

Carbs: 3g

Fiber: 1g

Net Carbs: 2g

Fat: 10g

Protein: 24g

Calories from:
Carbs: 4%
Fats: 46%
Protein: 49%

Ingredients:

- 1 pound ground turkey
- 1 yellow onion, chopped
- 3 cloves garlic, chopped
- 2 cups shredded mozzarella cheese
- 3 cups fresh spinach
- 2 teaspoons dried sage
- 1 teaspoon dried oregano
- Salt & black pepper, to taste
- Water

Directions:

1. Add all the ingredients minus the salt and black pepper to the base of a slow cooker and cover with about ¼ cup of water. Cook on high for 4 hours.

2. Season with salt and black pepper and serve.

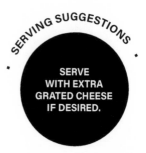

SERVING SUGGESTIONS

SERVE WITH EXTRA GRATED CHEESE IF DESIRED.

MEDIUM

Serves: 6

Prep Time: 10 minutes

Cook Time: 4 hours

Difficulty Level: 1

Cost: $$

Calories: 450
Carbs: 6g
Fiber: 1g
Net Carbs: 5g
Fat: 14g
Protein: 70g

Calories from:
Carbs: 5%
Fats: 30%
Protein: 66%

TOMATO VEGETABLE BEEF STEW (M)

Ingredients:

- 1 pound beef chuck, cubed
- 1 cup canned diced tomatoes
- 1 yellow onion, chopped
- tablespoons shallot, chopped
- 2 cloves garlic, chopped
- 1 carrot, chopped
- 1 cup kale, chopped
- 1 teaspoon dried thyme
- Salt & black pepper, to taste
- Water

Directions:

1. Add all the ingredients minus the salt and black pepper to the base of a slow cooker and cover with about ¼ cup of water. Cook on high for 4 hours.

2. Season with salt and black pepper and serve.

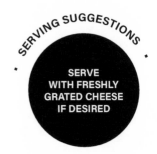

SERVING SUGGESTIONS

SERVE WITH FRESHLY GRATED CHEESE IF DESIRED

HAMBURGER BEEF STEW (M)

MEDIUM

Serves: 6

Prep Time: 10 minutes

Cook Time: 4 hours

Difficulty Level: 1

Cost: $

Calories: 324

Carbs: 7g

Fiber: 2g

Net Carbs: 5g

Fat: 18g

Protein: 34g

Calories from:
Carbs: 5%
Fats: 30%
Protein: 66%

Ingredients:

- 1 pound lean ground beef
- ¼ cup beef broth
- ½ cup tomato paste
- ½ cup canned diced tomatoes
- 1 yellow onion, chopped
- 2 cup shredded cheddar cheese
- 1 teaspoon Italian seasoning
- Salt & black pepper, to taste

Directions:

1. Add all the ingredients minus the salt and black pepper to the base of a slow cooker and cook on high for 4 hours.

2. Season with salt and black pepper and serve.

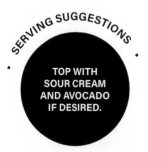

SERVING SUGGESTIONS

TOP WITH SOUR CREAM AND AVOCADO IF DESIRED.

AUTUMN HARVEST STEW (M)

MEDIUM

Serves: 6

Prep Time: 10 minutes

Cook Time: 4 hours

Difficulty Level: 1

Cost: $$

Calories: 457
Carbs: 8g
Fiber: 3g
Net Carbs: 5g
Fat: 14g
Protein: 70g

Calories from:
Carbs: 5%
Fats: 30%
Protein: 66%

Ingredients:

- 1 pound beef chuck, cubed
- ¼ cup beef broth
- ¼ cup balsamic vinegar
- 1 cup butternut squash, cubed
- 1 carrot, chopped
- 1 yellow onion, chopped
- 3 cloves garlic, chopped
- 1 cup kale, chopped
- 1 teaspoon dried thyme
- 1 teaspoon dried oregano
- 1 teaspoon dried sage
- Salt & black pepper, to taste

Directions:

1. Add all the ingredients minus the salt and black pepper to the base of a slow cooker and cook on high for 4 hours.

2. Season with salt and black pepper and serve.

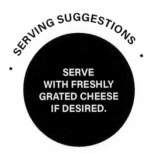

SERVING SUGGESTIONS

SERVE WITH FRESHLY GRATED CHEESE IF DESIRED.

Side Dishes

MEDIUM

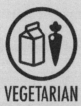

VEGETARIAN

Serves: 4

Prep Time: 15 minutes

Cook Time: 20 minutes

Difficulty Level: 2

Cost: $

Calories: 51

Carbs: 4g

Fiber: 1g

Net Carbs: 3g

Fat: 3g

Protein: 3g

Calories from:
Carbs: 24%
Fats: 53%
Protein: 24%

ZESTY ONION RINGS (V)(M)

Ingredients:

- 1 large onion, sliced into rings
- ½ cup almond flour
- 1 egg
- ½ teaspoon garlic powder
- 1 teaspoon paprika
- 1 teaspoon cayenne pepper
- 1 teaspoon salt

Directions:

1. Preheat the oven to 400°F, and line a baking sheet with parchment paper.

2. Add the egg to a mixing bowl, and then add the almond flour and seasoning to another bowl. Stir the almond flour mixture well.

3. Dip the sliced onions into the egg mixture, followed by the almond flour mix, covering both sides of the sliced onions.

4. Add the onion rings to the baking sheet and bake for about 10 minutes on each side or until crispy.

SERVING SUGGESTIONS

SERVE WITH YOUR FAVORITE KETO-FRIENDLY DIP.

HIGH

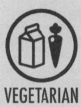

VEGETARIAN

Serves: 5

Prep Time: 5 minutes

Cook Time: 25 minutes

Difficulty Level: 2

Cost: $

Calories: 225

Carbs: 8g

Fiber: 4g

Net Carbs: 4g

Fat: 21g

Protein: 4g

Calories from:
Carbs: 7%
Fats: 86%
Protein: 7%

CARROT FRIES WITH HERB SAUCE (V)(H)

Ingredients:

Fries

- 5 carrots
- 1 tablespoon butter, melted
- 3 tablespoons olive oil
- Salt & pepper, to taste

Herb Sauce

- 5 tablespoon sour cream
- 5 tablespoon heavy cream
- 1 tablespoon fresh thyme, chopped
- 1 teaspoon fresh oregano, chopped
- ¼ teaspoon fresh rosemary, chopped
- 4 tablespoons Parmesan cheese, grated
- Salt & black pepper to taste

Directions:

1. Preheat the oven to 350°F. Prepare a baking sheet with parchment paper or nonstick cooking spray.

2. Cut the carrots into even pieces about the size of french fries.

continue in the next page ▶

CARROT FRIES WITH HERB SAUCE (V)(H)

HIGH

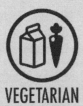

VEGETARIAN

Serves: 5

Prep Time: 5 minutes

Cook Time: 25 minutes

Difficulty Level: 2

Cost: $

Calories: 225

Carbs: 8g

Fiber: 4g

Net Carbs: 4g

Fat: 21g

Protein: 4g

Calories from:
Carbs: 7%
Fats: 86%
Protein: 7%

3. Place in a large mixing bowl and toss with the olive oil, melted butter, salt and black pepper. Transfer to the prepared baking sheet and bake for about 30 minutes, flipping halfway through.

4. While the carrots bake, prepare the herb sauce by combining the sour cream with the heavy cream, cheese and fresh herbs. Season with salt and black pepper to taste. Mix until smooth.

5. Remove the fries from the oven and serve alongside the herb sauce.

COOKING TIP

There's no need to peel the carrots. Wash them and cut them into fries with the skin still on.

As the herb sauce is better when served cold, prepare it in advance and refrigerate.

HIGH

Serves: 3

Prep Time: 15 minutes + chilling time

Cook Time: 15 minutes

Difficulty Level: 2

Cost: $$

Calories: 455

Carbs: 8g

Fiber: 5g

Net Carbs: 3g

Fat: 37g

Protein: 25g

Calories from:
Carbs: 3%
Fats: 75%
Protein: 22%

BACON & AVOCADO DEVILED EGGS (H)

Ingredients:

- 1 ripe avocado
- 4 large hard-boiled eggs
- 4 slices bacon, cooked and crumbled
- 1 red chili pepper, seeded and minced
- 1 garlic clove, minced
- 2 tablespoons lemon juice
- Salt & black pepper to taste

Directions:

1. Peel the eggs, halve them lengthwise and transfer the yolks to a mixing bowl.

2. Add the avocado, chili pepper, garlic and lemon juice to the bowl.

3. Mash with a fork until well combined. Season with salt and black pepper.

4. Scoop the mixture into the egg whites and top with the crumbled bacon.

5. Refrigerate until cold or serve right away.

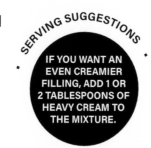

SERVING SUGGESTIONS

IF YOU WANT AN EVEN CREAMIER FILLING, ADD 1 OR 2 TABLESPOONS OF HEAVY CREAM TO THE MIXTURE.

HAM & CHEESE PIZZA ROLLS (H)

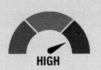

HIGH

Serves: 5

Prep Time: 15 minutes

Cook Time: 30 minutes

Difficulty Level: 2

Cost: $$

Calories: 492

Carbs: 6g

Fiber: 2g

Net Carbs: 4g

Fat: 35g

Protein: 35g

Calories from:
Carbs: 3%
Fats: 67%
Protein: 30%

Ingredients:

Dough

- ½ cup Parmesan cheese
- 1 cup mozzarella cheese
- 3 egg whites
- ¾ cup coconut flour
- 1 cup heavy cream

Filling

- 2 cups cooked ham, sliced
- 1 cup Gouda cheese, sliced
- 5 tablespoon tomato sauce
- 1 teaspoon crushed black pepper, for topping

Directions:

1. Preheat the oven to 400°F, and line a baking sheet with parchment paper.

2. In a food processor, combine the ingredients for the crust and process until a smooth dough forms. You may need to add water, a tablespoon at a time, to achieve this result.

3. Flatten the dough into a rectangular shape onto the prepared baking sheet. Bake for about 15 minutes. Remove from the oven and allow to cool slightly.

Serves: 5

Prep Time: 5 minutes

Cook Time: 25 minutes

Difficulty Level: 2

Cost: $

Calories: 492

Carbs: 6g

Fiber: 2g

Net Carbs: 4g

Fat: 35g

Protein: 35g

Calories from:
Carbs: 3%
Fats: 67%
Protein: 30%

4. Spread the tomato sauce evenly across the dough. Top with the sliced ham and Gouda cheese.

5. Roll the dough carefully into a log. Slice the log into 5 even pieces and place each one back onto the baking sheet. Sprinkle with crushed black pepper.

6. Bake again for about 10 minutes until the dough is golden brown and the cheese is bubbly.

COOKING TIP

After the first baking, the dough should be soft but dry. Wait for the dough to cool down a bit before rolling as this helps prevent the dough from falling apart.

Bisques, Chowders and Broths

LOBSTER BISQUE (M)

MEDIUM

Serves: 6

Prep Time: 10 minutes

Cook Time: 13-15 minutes

Difficulty Level: 1

Cost: $$

Calories: 187
Carbs: 6g
Fiber: 1g
Net Carbs: 5g
Fat: 11g
Protein: 15g

Calories from:
Carbs: 11%
Fats: 55%
Protein: 34%

Ingredients:

- ¾ pound cooked lobster, chopped
- 4 cups chicken broth
- 1 cup heavy cream
- 1 can (14.5 ounces) diced tomatoes
- 1 yellow onion, chopped
- 2 cloves garlic, chopped
- ½ teaspoon paprika
- ½ teaspoon salt
- ¼ teaspoon black pepper
- 1 tablespoon coconut oil, for cooking

Directions:

1. Add the coconut oil to a stockpot over medium heat.

2. Sauté the garlic and onion for 3 to 5 minutes.

3. Add the chicken broth, diced tomatoes and spices and bring to a boil.

4. Reduce to a simmer, and simmer for 10 minutes.

5. Warm the heavy cream, and then add to the soup.

6. Use an immersion blender and blend the soup until creamy.

7. Stir in the cooked lobster and serve.

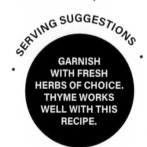

SERVING SUGGESTIONS

GARNISH WITH FRESH HERBS OF CHOICE. THYME WORKS WELL WITH THIS RECIPE.

93

WHITE CLAM CHOWDER (M)

MEDIUM

Serves: 10

Prep Time: 10 minutes

Cook Time: 6 hours

Difficulty Level: 1

Cost: $$

Calories: 110

Carbs: 5g

Fiber: 0g

Net Carbs: 5

Fat: 6g

Protein: 11g

Calories from:
Carbs: 17%
Fats: 46%
Protein: 37%

Ingredients:

- 20 ounces canned whole baby clams, drained
- ¼ cup reduced sodium chicken broth
- 2 cups water
- 1 cup heavy cream
- ½ cup whipped cream cheese
- 1 sweet onion, chopped
- 1 shallot, chopped
- 2 cloves garlic, chopped
- 1 teaspoon thyme
- 1 teaspoon salt
- ¼ teaspoon black pepper

Directions:

1. Add all the ingredients minus the heavy cream and cream cheese to the base of a slow cooker. Cook on low for 6 hours.

2. Warm the heavy cream, and then whisk in the cream cheese and warmed cream until smooth.

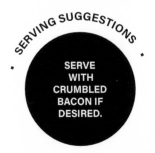

SERVING SUGGESTIONS

SERVE WITH CRUMBLED BACON IF DESIRED.

MUSHROOM & BACON CHOWDER (H)

HIGH

Serves: 6

Prep Time: 10 minutes

Cook Time: 4 hours

Difficulty Level: 1

Cost: $$

Calories: 373

Carbs: 5g

Fiber: 1g

Net Carbs: 4g

Fat: 32g

Protein: 16g

Calories from:
Carbs: 4%
Fats: 78%
Protein: 17%

Ingredients:

- 3 cups chicken broth
- 1 cup heavy cream
- 1 cup whipped cream cheese
- 1 cup cremini mushrooms
- 8 slices bacon, chopped
- 1 yellow onion, chopped
- 2 cloves garlic, chopped
- 1 teaspoon freshly chopped thyme
- Salt & black pepper, to taste

Directions:

1. Add all the ingredients minus the heavy cream and cream cheese to the base of a slow cooker. Cook on low for 4 hours.

2. Warm the heavy cream, and then whisk in the cream cheese and warmed cream until smooth.

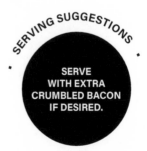

SERVING SUGGESTIONS

SERVE WITH EXTRA CRUMBLED BACON IF DESIRED.

CAULIFLOWER MAC & CHEESE CHOWDER (H)

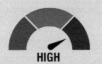

HIGH

Serves: 4

Prep Time: 10 minutes

Cook Time: 4 hours

Difficulty Level: 1

Cost: $$

Calories: 266

Carbs: 6g

Fiber: 2g

Net Carbs: 4g

Fat: 22g

Protein: 13g

Calories from:
Carbs: 6%
Fats: 74%
Protein: 20%

Ingredients:

- 1 cauliflower head, cut into florets
- 3 cups chicken broth
- 1 cup heavy cream
- 1 cup shredded cheddar cheese
- 2 cloves garlic, chopped
- 1 teaspoon freshly chopped thyme
- Salt & black pepper, to taste

Directions:

1. Add all the ingredients minus the heavy cream and shredded cheese to the base of a slow cooker. Cook on low for 4 hours.

2. Warm the heavy cream, and then whisk in the warmed cream and cheese until smooth.

3. Use an immersion blender and blend until creamy and smooth.

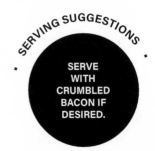

SERVING SUGGESTIONS

SERVE WITH CRUMBLED BACON IF DESIRED.

CHICKEN BONE BROTH USING THE INSTANT POT (L)

LOW

Serves: 6

Prep Time: 10 minutes

Cook Time: 120 minutes

Difficulty Level: 1

Cost: $$

Calories: 19

Carbs: 4g

Fiber: 1g

Net Carbs: 3g

Fat: 0g

Protein: 1g

Calories from:
Carbs: 75%
Fats: 0%
Protein: 25%

Ingredients:

- Bones from a 4-pound chicken
- 1 yellow onion, quartered
- 4 garlic cloves
- 1 large carrot, halved
- 2 stalks celery, halved
- 1 bay leaf
- 1 tablespoon raw apple cider vinegar
- 1 large pinch of salt
- 4 black peppercorns
- Fresh water

Directions:

1. Add all the ingredients to the base of the Instant pot and cover with enough water to cover the bones and vegetables.

2. Place the lid on the Instant Pot and make sure the valve is set to sealing.

3. Select manual and set to 120 minutes.

4. Once the timer goes off, allow the pressure to release naturally. Allow the broth to sit out and cool.

5. Strain the broth into glass jars and freeze or refrigerate.

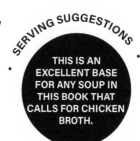

SERVING SUGGESTIONS

THIS IS AN EXCELLENT BASE FOR ANY SOUP IN THIS BOOK THAT CALLS FOR CHICKEN BROTH.

BEEF BONE BROTH USING THE INSTANT POT (L)

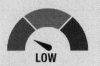

LOW

Serves: 6

Prep Time: 10 minutes

Cook Time: 120 minutes

Difficulty Level: 1

Cost: $$

Calories: 19

Carbs: 4g

Fiber: 1g

Net Carbs: 3g

Fat: 0g

Protein: 1g

Calories from:
Carbs: 75%
Fats: 0%
Protein: 25%

Ingredients:

- 2 pounds assorted beef bones
- 1 yellow onion, quartered
- 4 garlic cloves
- 1 large carrot, halved
- 2 stalks celery, halved
- 1 bay leaf
- 2 sprigs rosemary
- 2 sprigs thyme
- 1 tablespoon raw apple cider vinegar
- 1 large pinch of salt
- 4 black peppercorns
- Fresh water

Directions:

1. Add all the ingredients to the base of the Instant pot and cover with enough water to cover the bones and vegetables.

2. Place the lid on the Instant Pot and make sure the valve is set to sealing.

3. Select manual and set to 120 minutes.

4. Once the timer goes off, allow the pressure to release naturally. Allow the broth to sit out and cool.

5. Strain the broth into glass jars and freeze or refrigerate.

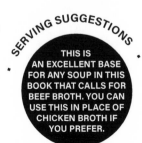

SERVING SUGGESTIONS

THIS IS AN EXCELLENT BASE FOR ANY SOUP IN THIS BOOK THAT CALLS FOR BEEF BROTH. YOU CAN USE THIS IN PLACE OF CHICKEN BROTH IF YOU PREFER.

VEGETABLE BROTH USING THE INSTANT POT (V)(L)

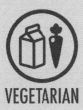

VEGETARIAN

Serves: 8

Prep Time: 10 minutes

Cook Time: 120 minutes

Difficulty Level: 1

Cost: $$

Calories: 27

Carbs: 6g

Fiber: 2g

Net Carbs: 4g

Fat: 0g

Protein: 1g

Calories from:
Carbs: 80%
Fats: 0%
Protein: 20%

Ingredients:

* 1 cup mixed frozen vegetables
* 1 onion, quartered
* 2 stalks celery, chopped
* 2 carrots, chopped
* 3 garlic cloves, chopped
* 1 bay leaf
* 2 sprigs rosemary
* 2 sprigs thyme
* 1 large pinch of salt
* 4 black peppercorns
* 8 cups water

Directions:

1. Add all the ingredients to the base of the Instant Pot.

2. Place the lid on the Instant Pot and make sure the valve is set to sealing.

3. Select manual and set to 120 minutes.

4. Once the timer goes off, allow the pressure to release naturally. Allow the broth to sit out and cool.

5. Strain the broth into glass jars and freeze or refrigerate.

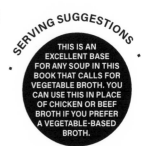

SERVING SUGGESTIONS

THIS IS AN EXCELLENT BASE FOR ANY SOUP IN THIS BOOK THAT CALLS FOR VEGETABLE BROTH. YOU CAN USE THIS IN PLACE OF CHICKEN OR BEEF BROTH IF YOU PREFER A VEGETABLE-BASED BROTH.

Soup Bread

HIGH

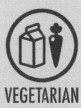

VEGETARIAN

Serves: 3

Prep Time: 15 minutes

Cook Time: 20 minutes

Difficulty Level: 1

Cost: $

Calories: 300

Carbs: 10g

Fiber: 5g

Net Carbs: 5g

Fat: 23g

Protein: 16g

Calories from:
Carbs: 7%
Fats: 72%
Protein: 21%

ROSEMARY & THYME FLAT BREAD (V)(H)

Ingredients:

- ½ cup almond flour
- 8 large egg whites
- 1 ½ teaspoon gluten-free baking powder
- 2 teaspoons fresh thyme, chopped
- ¼ teaspoon ground turmeric
- 3 tablespoons fresh rosemary, chopped
- 2 tablespoons olive oil
- ¼ teaspoon salt

Directions:

1. In a blender or food processor, combine all of the ingredients except for the olive oil and blend until well combined.

2. In a large frying pan, heat about a third of the olive oil over medium heat.

3. Pour one-third of the mixture into the frying pan and allow to cook for about 3 minutes until bubbles start to appear. Flip carefully and continue cooking for an additional 3 minutes.

4. Remove the flatbread from the pan and repeat with the remaining batter.

SERVING SUGGESTIONS

SERVE WITH ONE OF YOUR FAVORITE SOUPS OR STEWS FROM THIS BOOK.

MEDIUM

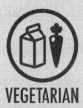

VEGETARIAN

Serves: 10

Prep Time: 10 minutes

Cook Time: 20 minutes

Difficulty Level: 1

Cost: $$

Calories: 194

Carbs: 8g

Fiber: 3g

Net Carbs: 5g

Fat: 17g

Protein: 6g

Calories from:
Carbs: 10%
Fats: 78%
Protein: 12%

DINNER ROLLS
(V)(M)

Ingredients:

- 6 eggs, separated
- ½ cup coconut flour
- ¼ cup psyllium husk (whole husk including seeds)
- 1 tablespoon garlic powder
- ½ teaspoon salt
- 1 teaspoon apple cider vinegar
- 6 tablespoons butter
- 1 ½ teaspoons baking powder

Directions:

1. Preheat the oven to 350°F, and line a baking sheet with parchment paper.

2. Cream the butter, and add in 1 egg yolk at a time, placing the egg whites into a separate bowl.

3. Add the remaining ingredients to the butter and egg mixture, and mix until combined. Set aside.

4. Whip the egg whites with a stand mixer or a handheld mixer until stiff peaks form. Fold the butter mix into the egg whites. Mix until just combined.

5. Shape into 10 rolls, and bake for 20 minutes. Serve warm.

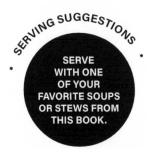

SERVING SUGGESTIONS

SERVE WITH ONE OF YOUR FAVORITE SOUPS OR STEWS FROM THIS BOOK.

MEDIUM

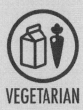

VEGETARIAN

Serves: 13 (1 breadstick each)

Prep Time: 10 minutes

Cook Time: 20 minutes

Difficulty Level: 1

Cost: $$

Calories: 47
Carbs: 2g
Fiber: 1g
Net Carbs: 1g
Fat: 3g
Protein: 16g

Calories from:
Carbs: 4%
Fats: 28%
Protein: 67%

CHEESY BREADSTICKS (V)(M)

Ingredients:

- 2 cups shredded mozzarella cheese
- 2 tablespoons coconut flour
- 2 eggs
- 1 pinch of salt

Toppings:

- ½ cup shredded Parmesan cheese
- 1 tablespoon Italian seasoning
- ½ teaspoon garlic powder

Directions:

1. Preheat the oven to 350° F, and line a baking sheet with parchment paper.

2. Add the mozzarella cheese, coconut flour, eggs and salt to a food processor and process until smooth.

3. Scoop the mixture onto the lined baking sheet and flatten to about 1-inch thick, forming a square.

4. Bake for 15 minutes.

5. Remove from the oven and sprinkle with the Parmesan cheese, Italian seasoning and garlic powder.

6. Bake for an additional 5 minutes or until the Parmesan cheese is melted.

7. Remove from the oven and allow the breadsticks to cool for 10 to 15 minutes before slicing into sticks.

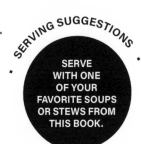

SERVING SUGGESTIONS

SERVE WITH ONE OF YOUR FAVORITE SOUPS OR STEWS FROM THIS BOOK.

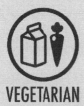

VEGETARIAN

Serves: 3

Prep Time: 15 minutes

Cook Time: 20 minutes

Difficulty Level: 1

Cost: $

Calories: 50

Carbs: 0g

Fiber: 0g

Net Carbs: 0g

Fat: 5g

Protein: 2g

Calories from:
Carbs: 0%
Fats: 85%
Protein: 15%

CLOUD BREAD
(V)(H)

Ingredients:

- 3 eggs, separated
- 3 tablespoons butter
- ¼ teaspoon apple cider vinegar
- 1 drop stevia extract
- ½ teaspoon baking powder
- 1 pinch of salt

Directions:

1. Preheat the oven to 300°F, and line a baking sheet with parchment paper.

2. Place the egg yolks in one bowl and the egg whites in another. In the bowl with the yolks, whisk the eggs and add the remaining ingredients.

3. Whip the egg whites with a stand or handheld mixer until stiff peaks form. Fold the egg yolk mixture into the egg whites and combine gently.

4. Form into 10 rounds, and place on the baking sheet.

5. Bake for about 30 minutes or until golden brown.

6. Serve warm, and store the leftovers covered in the refrigerator.

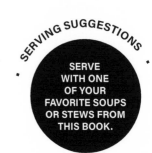

SERVING SUGGESTIONS

SERVE WITH ONE OF YOUR FAVORITE SOUPS OR STEWS FROM THIS BOOK.

Soup Seasonings & Toppings

LOW

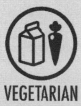

VEGETARIAN

Serves: 6

Prep Time: 10 minutes

Cook Time: None

Difficulty Level: 1

Cost: $

Calories: 10

Carbs: 2g

Fiber: 1g

Net Carbs: 1g

Fat: 0g

Protein: 0g

Calories from:
Carbs: 100%
Fats: 0%
Protein: 0%

MULTI-HERB BLEND (V)(L)

Ingredients:

- 1 tablespoon oregano
- 1 tablespoon thyme
- 1 teaspoon dried rosemary
- 2 teaspoons garlic powder
- 1 teaspoon onion powder
- 1 teaspoon cracked black pepper
- ½ teaspoon sea salt

Directions:

1. Add all the spices to a mixing bowl and whisk well.

2. Pour into a glass jar and store in the pantry.

3. Be sure to label your spice mix.

SERVING SUGGESTIONS

THIS SEASONING MIX GOES WELL WITH ANY OF THE SOUP RECIPES THAT CALL FOR CHICKEN OR TURKEY. SWAP OUT THE SEASONING THAT IS CALLED FOR IN THE RECIPE AND ADD 1 TO 2 TEASPOONS OF THIS MIX INSTEAD.

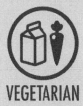

VEGETARIAN

Serves: 6

Prep Time: 10 minutes

Cook Time: None

Difficulty Level: 1

Cost: $

Calories: 6
Carbs: 1g
Fiber: 1g
Net Carbs: 0g
Fat: 0g
Protein: 0g

Calories from:
Carbs: 100%
Fats: 0%
Protein: 0%

NUTMEG & CLOVE SPICE MIX (V)(L)

Ingredients:

- 1 tablespoon ground cinnamon
- 1 teaspoon ground nutmeg
- 1 teaspoon ground cloves
- ½ teaspoon sea salt

Directions:

1. Add all the spices to a mixing bowl and whisk well.

2. Pour into a glass jar and store in the pantry.

3. Be sure to label your spice mix.

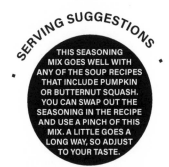

SERVING SUGGESTIONS

THIS SEASONING MIX GOES WELL WITH ANY OF THE SOUP RECIPES THAT INCLUDE PUMPKIN OR BUTTERNUT SQUASH. YOU CAN SWAP OUT THE SEASONING IN THE RECIPE AND USE A PINCH OF THIS MIX. A LITTLE GOES A LONG WAY, SO ADJUST TO YOUR TASTE.

LOW

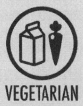

VEGETARIAN

Serves: 6

Prep Time: 10 minutes

Cook Time: None

Difficulty Level: 1

Cost: $

Calories: 8
Carbs: 2g
Fiber: 1g
Net Carbs: 1g
Fat: 0g
Protein: 0g

Calories from:
Carbs: 100%
Fats: 0%
Protein: 0%

LEMON PEPPER SPICE MIX (V)(L)

Ingredients:

- 1 tablespoon lemon zest
- 2 tablespoons cracked black pepper
- 1 teaspoon garlic powder
- ½ teaspoon sea salt

Directions:

1. Add all the spices to a mixing bowl and whisk well.

2. Pour into a glass jar and store in the pantry.

3. Be sure to label your spice mix.

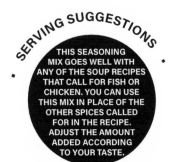

SERVING SUGGESTIONS

THIS SEASONING MIX GOES WELL WITH ANY OF THE SOUP RECIPES THAT CALL FOR FISH OR CHICKEN. YOU CAN USE THIS MIX IN PLACE OF THE OTHER SPICES CALLED FOR IN THE RECIPE. ADJUST THE AMOUNT ADDED ACCORDING TO YOUR TASTE.

LOW

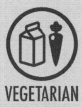

VEGETARIAN

Serves: 6

Prep Time: 10 minutes

Cook Time: None

Difficulty Level: 1

Cost: $

Calories: 11
Carbs: 2g
Fiber: 1g
Net Carbs: 1g
Fat: 0g
Protein: 0g

Calories from:
Carbs: 100%
Fats: 0%
Protein: 0%

SPICY CAJUN SEASONING (V)(L)

Ingredients:

- 1 teaspoon paprika
- 1 teaspoon cayenne pepper
- 1 teaspoon chili powder
- 1 teaspoon dried thyme
- 1 teaspoon dried oregano
- 2 teaspoons garlic powder
- 2 teaspoons onion powder
- 1 teaspoon cracked black pepper
- ½ teaspoon sea salt

Directions:

1. Add all the spices to a mixing bowl and whisk well.

2. Pour into a glass jar and store in the pantry.

3. Be sure to label your spice mix.

SERVING SUGGESTIONS

THIS SEASONING MIX GOES WELL WITH ANY OF THE SPICY SOUP RECIPES. YOU CAN USE THIS MIX IN PLACE OF THE OTHER SPICES CALLED FOR IN THE RECIPE. ADJUST THE AMOUNT ADDED ACCORDING TO YOUR TASTE.

Made in the USA
Monee, IL
24 April 2021

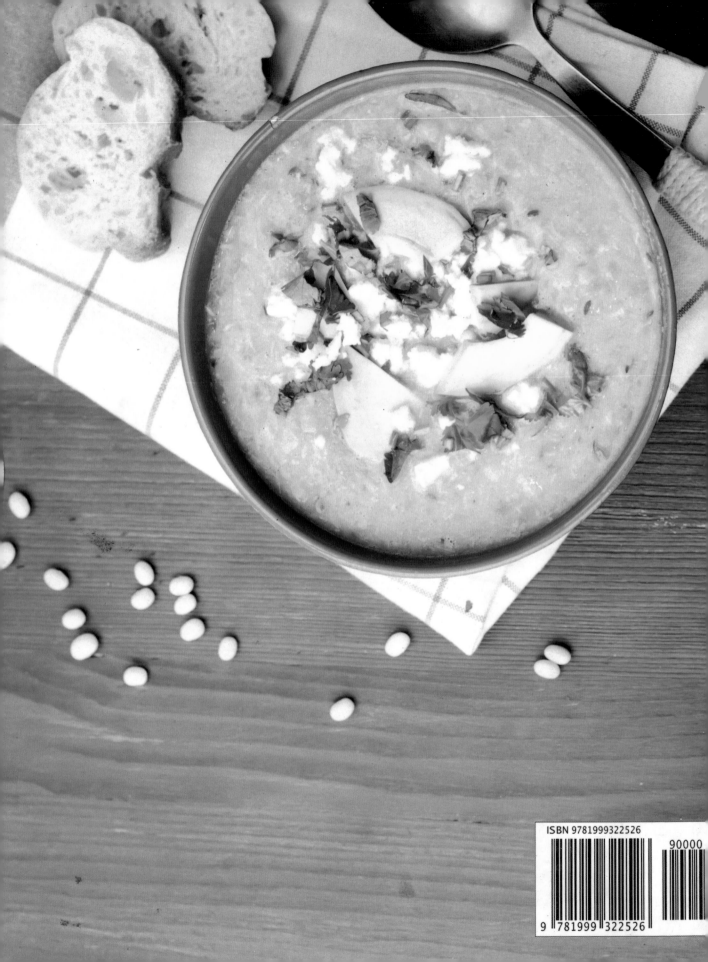

ISBN 9781999322526

90000

9 781999 322526